Stroke

Date: 1/23/18

616.81 STR
Stroke /

What Do I Do Now?

SERIES CO-EDITORS-IN-CHIEF

Lawrence C. Newman, MD
Director of the Headache Institute
Department of Neurology
St. Luke's-Roosevelt Hospital Center
New York, New York

Morris Levin, MD
Co-director of the Dartmouth Headache Center
Director of the Dartmouth Neurology Residency Training Program
Section of Neurology
Dartmouth Hitchcock Medical Center
Lebanon, New Hampshire

Stroke

SECOND EDITION

Louis R. Caplan, MD, FACP, FAAN
Professor of Neurology
Harvard Medical School
Beth Israel Deaconess Medical Center
Boston, MA

Vasileios-Arsenios Lioutas, MD
Instructor of Neurology
Harvard Medical School
Division of Cerebrovascular Diseases
Beth Israel Deaconess Medical Center
Boston, MA

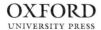

OXFORD
UNIVERSITY PRESS

OXFORD
UNIVERSITY PRESS

Oxford University Press is a department of the University of Oxford. It furthers
the University's objective of excellence in research, scholarship, and education
by publishing worldwide. Oxford is a registered trade mark of Oxford University
Press in the UK and certain other countries.

Published in the United States of America by Oxford University Press
198 Madison Avenue, New York, NY 10016, United States of America.

Library of Congress Cataloging-in-Publication Data
Names: Caplan, Louis R., editor. | Lioutas, Vasileios-Arsenios, editor.
Title: Stroke / [edited by] Louis R. Caplan, Vasileios-Arsenios Lioutas.
Other titles: Stroke (Caplan) | What do I do now?
Description: Second edition. | Oxford ; New York : Oxford University Press, 2016. |
Series: What do I do now? | Includes bibliographical references and index.
Identifiers: LCCN 2015042321 | ISBN 9780190497255 (pbk. : alk. paper)
Subjects: | MESH: Stroke—diagnosis—Case Reports. | Stroke—therapy—Case Reports.
Classification: LCC RC388.5 | NLM WL 356 | DDC 616.8/1—dc23
LC record available at http://lccn.loc.gov/2015042321

9 8 7 6 5 4 3 2 1
Printed by Webcom, Canada

Contents

Preface

C. Miller Fisher's aphorism, that one learns neurology "stroke by stroke," is probably all too familiar to most neurologists by now, but it is more than just a clever quote. If an aphorism is, in Karl Kraus's words, either a half-truth or a truth and a half, then it certainly errs on the side of the latter. Historically, clinicopathologic observations of stroke-related brain lesions and the loss of function of the affected areas were the main source of information on the normal function of these areas. Even in the current era of abundantly available diagnostic imaging, diagnosis and anatomic localization of stroke symptoms and syndromes remain critical, and they can be an excellent window into clinical neuroanatomy for medical students and neurology residents. Acute stroke management and secondary prevention have been revolutionized during the past two decades, which makes stroke a lot more exciting and complex than a simple exercise in applied neuroanatomy.

Stroke is a heterogeneous disease and a detailed, comprehensive review would exceed the scope of this book. Our goal is dual: to highlight how intriguing the diagnostic process can be in real-life encounters and to offer management insight that, hopefully, proves helpful for the practicing clinician. In an effort to make the read more engaging, we made several changes from the first edition. Instead of refining the cases discussed in the first edition, we replaced most of them with new ones. Readers are challenged with a mixture of bread-and-butter cases, and more peculiar and idiosyncratic ones. Although the first kind is encountered more frequently, the latter spark the imagination and can be a perfect antidote to the mental fatigue brought by a grueling, long day at work in the middle of a Boston winter. We also made changes in the format, avoiding disclosure of the diagnosis until the discussion, in an effort to challenge readers to think diagnostically. Chapter titles have been left intentionally vague so as not to give away the diagnoses and, although they range from the prosaic to the more creative, readers will realize they are not chosen thoughtlessly. We have added several references for further reading at the end of each chapter and we hope they help readers to delve further into the details and implications of the case at hand.

All chapter authors are currently members of the Beth Israel Deaconess Medical Center Neurology Department or have trained in our Stroke Fellowship with us. We reviewed and edited all cases carefully for a minimum of uniformity of dialectic style, but we mostly allowed for variations in narrative-style individuality. We hope this adds to the appeal of the book and makes it more direct and enjoyable.

Boston, December 2015
Louis R. Caplan
Vasileios-Arsenios Lioutas

Contributors

Elorm Avakame, BS
Harvard Medical School
Boston, MA

Marc Bouffard, MD
Beth Israel Deaconess
Medical Center
Harvard Medical School
Boston, MA

Merritt W. Brown, MD
University of Pennsylvania
Philadelphia, PA

Louis R. Caplan, MD,
FACP, FAAN
Harvard Medical School
Beth Israel Deaconess
Medical Center
Boston, MA

Luciana Catanese, MD
Beth Israel Deaconess
Medical Center
Harvard Medical School
Boston, MA

Bart Chwalisz, MD
Massachusetts General Hospital
Harvard Medical School
Boston, MA

Sourabh Lahoti, MD
University of Kentucky
Medical Center
Lexington, KY

Lester Y. Leung, MD
Department of Neurology
Tufts Medical Center
Boston, MA

Vasileios-Arsenios Lioutas, MD
Harvard Medical School
Department of Neurology
Beth Israel Deaconess
Medical Center
Boston, MA

Mark McAllister, MD
Saint Elizabeth Hospital
Boston, MA

D. Eric Searls, MD
Beth Israel Deaconess
Medical Center
Harvard Medical School
Boston, MA

Shruti Sonni, MD
Cambridge Health Alliance
Beth Israel Deaconess
Medical Center
Harvard Medical School
Boston, MA

Meg Van Nostrand, MD
Beth Israel Deaconess
Medical Center
Harvard Medical School
Boston, MA

1 Confused after a Nap

Vasileios-Arsenios Lioutas

An 80-year-old left-handed woman developed
acute-onset left-sided temporal throbbing
headache. She has a history of migraines and
initially considered this to be a migraine attack,
with the exception that the headache onset was
unusually abrupt. After a short nap, her headache
was somewhat better, but she exhibited odd
behaviors, which were described by her family
members as confusion, dysarthric speech, and
difficulty handling commonly used utensils, such as
the phone, which she was holding upside down and
eventually dropped.

   Besides migraines, the patient has a history of
anxiety, and some recent episodes of confusion
and disorientation that were interpreted as
manifestations of her anxiety. Her only medications
include pantoprazole and alprazolam as needed for
anxiety.

   On examination 3 hours after symptom onset,
the patient's blood pressure is 135/60, and her pulse

is 82 and regular. Her heart is not enlarged. She is alert and attends to the examiner. She does not follow any commands, but is able to speak fluently with clear articulation, although the content of her speech is nonsensical. Her gaze is conjugate and her pupils equal, round, and reactive to light. She does not have any focal weakness, although her motor examination is limited by her inability to cooperate fully.

Basic laboratory test results, including complete blood count, chemistry, and coagulation panel, are unremarkable.

What do you do now?

LOBAR INTRACEREBRAL HEMORRHAGE RESULTING FROM AMYLOID ANGIOPATHY

Discussion Questions

1. What is the differential diagnosis?
2. What imaging study should be performed?
3. What should be the immediate care? Is there a role for surgical intervention?
4. What additional workup is necessary and what are the potential causes?

Discussion

A first important point is the discordance between collateral history as provided by family members and the findings on examination, which often can be misleading. Aphasia can be described under several nonspecific terms: confusion, bizarre behavior, or difficulty speaking. It is therefore very important for the clinician to inquire about the details and specifics of the presentation, and to perform a thorough examination. The patient's examination is suggestive of fluent aphasia (traditionally also known as *Wernicke's aphasia*), which is much more accurately localizing than dysarthria or nonspecific confusion.

Given the history of benzodiazepine use and migraine, alprazolam overdose or withdrawal and confusional migraine should be considered in the differential diagnosis. However, symptom duration and the localizing sign of fluent aphasia make the first unlikely, whereas the atypical rate of onset and nature of headache raise suspicion for an alternative etiology. Given the presence of headache, intracranial hemorrhage should be considered. Headache is uncommon in ischemic stroke, although the possibility of carotid artery dissection should be in the clinician's radar. In this case, there is no history of head or neck trauma that would predispose the patient to carotid dissection. The combination of headache and symptom laterality can often guide the clinician, although in this particular case the fact that the patient is left-handed does not allow safe assumptions regarding hemisphere dominance. An imaging study is necessary.

On an urgent basis, a noncontrast head CT is the imaging study of choice. It is brief, easily tolerated, and does not expose patients to contrast load. CT results are shown in Figure 1.1a.

This patient has a left temporal hematoma. She should be monitored closely, with frequent neurological assessments, to detect and intervene on deterioration as early as possible. Decrease in the level of consciousness, enlargement of the left pupil, a new appearance of a gaze palsy, or Babinski sign would indicate increased pressure within the left temporal lobe. Hematoma expansion and clinical deterioration tend to occur within the first hours of the index event. Additional immediate concerns for the clinician include reversal of possible coagulopathy and blood pressure control, both of which should be addressed as expeditiously as possible. In the case of thrombocytopenia, platelet transfusion should be administered to restore the platelet count to more than100,000; vitamin K and fresh-frozen plasma or prothrombin complex concentrate should be given for a target international normalized ratio of 1.4 or less. Antithrombotic medications should be held.

The relation of blood pressure to outcome is more complex than anticipated initially. It is thought to be a major factor in contributing to hematoma growth and poor functional outcome, and although two major trials failed to meet the efficacy endpoint (Intensive Blood Pressure Reduction in Acute Cerebral Hemorrhage Trial [INTERACT] and INTERACT-2), its safety and feasibility were proved and a trend toward better outcome was observed. The current standard of care mandates that systolic blood

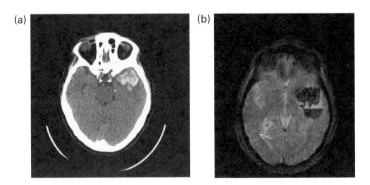

FIGURE 1.1 (a) Noncontrast head CT with left anterior lobar hemorrhage. (b) Gradient echo MRI sequence indicating left temporal hematoma and one cortical microbleed (arrow).

pressure should be lowered to less than 140 mm Hg. Agents of choice commonly include intermittent intravenous labetalol or hydralazine infusions, although in situations when a closer titration is necessary, continuous nicardipine infusion is preferred. Despite its rapid blood pressure-lowering effect, nitroprusside should be avoided in such patients because it increases intracranial pressure.

Surgical hematoma evacuation in supratentorial hemorrhages remains controversial. Despite its anticipated benefit, two randomized trials failed to demonstrate this. As a result, surgical hematoma evacuation is offered as rescue therapy on a patient-by-patient basis in cases of early deterioration.

The differential diagnosis in intracerebral hemorrhage (ICH) is broad, but common causes include hypertensive hemorrhage, amyloid angiopathy, underlying mass, or vascular lesion. In the proper context, cerebral venous thrombosis or hemorrhagic conversion of an ischemic infarct should be considered as well. In this patient, her normal blood pressure, and her age and lobar localization make cerebral amyloid angiopathy by far the most likely diagnosis.

A vascular study would be useful; CT angiography can be performed quickly and its sensitivity is high. If performed early, it offers the additional benefit of identifying patients at risk for hematoma expansion through the so-called "spot sign" (nidus of contrast extravasation thought to represent active hemorrhage). Brain MRI can help identify underlying structural lesions such as primary or metastatic hemorrhagic tumors and, most importantly, can identify cerebral microbleeds, which are blood degradation products in close proximity to abnormal vessels and constitute the imaging hallmark of underlying amyloid angiopathy if located within the lobar regions. In this case, the lobar location of the hemorrhage and the presence of additional cerebral microbleeds in a lobar location (Figure 1.1b) strongly suggest that the underlying etiology of this hemorrhage is amyloid angiopathy.

KEY POINTS TO REMEMBER

- Ischemic stroke and ICH can be difficult to distinguish clinically, but the presence of headache makes hemorrhage more likely.

- No directed treatments for ICH are available, but close monitoring, blood pressure management, and coagulopathy reversal are important parameters of acute ICH management.
- Neuroimaging, especially brain MRI, can provide key information regarding hemorrhage etiology.
- Lobar location of a primary hemorrhage suggests amyloid angiopathy, whereas a nonlobar location is more likely to be secondary to hypertension.
- Cortical microbleeds seen on MRI suggest an underlying amyloid angiopathy as the most likely explanation.

Further Reading

Anderson CS, Heeley E, Huang Y et al. Rapid blood-pressure lowering in patients with acute intracerebral hemorrhage. *N Engl J Med*. 2013;368:2355–2365.

Greenberg SM, Vernooij MW, Cordonnier C, et al. Cerebral microbleeds: a guide to detection and interpretation. *Lancet Neurol*. 2009;8(2):165–174.

Hemphill JC 3rd, Greenberg SM, Anderson CS et al. Guidelines for the management of spontaneous intracerebral hemorrhage: a guideline for healthcare professionals. From the American Heart Association/American Stroke Association. *Stroke*. 2015;46(7):2032–2060.

Mendelow AD, Gregson BA, Rowan EN, Murray GD, Gholkar A, Mitchell PM; STICH II Investigators Early surgery versus initial conservative treatment in patients with spontaneous supratentorial lobar intracerebral haematomas (STICH II): a randomised trial. *Lancet*. 2013;382(9890):397–408.

Headache after a Beach Trip

Mark McAllister

A 34-year-old woman presents to the emergency
department with severe headache that has lasted
2 days. The headache began gradually, and it
is described as posterior and throbbing. When
questioned, the patient indicates accompanying
numbness in the left face and arm without
associated weakness, speech changes, dizziness,
and vision changes. The pain is increasing
progressively. There is no antecedent trauma, and
headaches are not typical for her. The patient notes
that acetaminophen was ineffective as pain relief.
The day before onset she reports lying on the beach
without strenuous activity. She admits to little fluid
intake that day. The patient has a past medical
history of hypothyroidism and tobacco dependency
(one pack per day). Her home medications are
levothyroxine and an estrogen-containing oral
contraceptive. Her heart rate is 96 and regular, and
her blood pressure is 128/78. Examination is notable

for decreased pinprick and light touch over the right face and arm, sparing the leg. The remainder of the neurological examination is normal.

What do you do now?

CEREBRAL VENOUS SINUS THROMBOSIS

Discussion Questions

1. What are possible etiologies?
2. What imaging studies would you pursue?
3. What would be your treatment of choice?

Discussion

In this previously healthy woman presenting with headache, there are several concerning aspects to her symptoms. That the headache is new for the patient and it has a relentlessly progressive course require investigation. In addition, focal neurological signs always warrant further consideration.

The differential diagnosis includes migraine, tension-type headache, idiopathic intracranial hypertension, subarachnoid hemorrhage, subdural or epidural hematoma, intracerebral hemorrhage (ICH), arterial dissection or thromboembolism, reversible cerebral vasoconstriction syndrome, and cerebral venous sinus thrombosis (CVST). Diagnoses of subarachnoid hemorrhage, reversible cerebral vasoconstriction syndrome, arterial dissection or thromboembolism, and ICH are more typically characterized by sudden-onset headache. In addition, the patient denies trauma, which usually precedes subdural or epidural hematomas. She does have thrombotic risk factors of smoking, hormonal birth control, and dehydration. It is prudent to inquire about other thrombotic risk factors such as previous deep vein thrombosis, pulmonary embolism, spontaneous abortion, inflammatory conditions, and pregnancy/puerperium.

Given the differential diagnosis, neuroimaging is indicated. Noncontrast CT of the head is normal. Brain MRI demonstrates restricted diffusion in the right temporal/parietal lobes with evidence of surrounding edema on T2-weighted images. A magnetic resonance venogram reveals occlusion of the right transverse and sigmoid sinuses with extension to the jugular vein, confirming the diagnosis of CVST.

The typical patient with CVST is female and young, with an average age of about 36 years. Inciting factors include pregnancy/puerperium, hormonal birth control, hypercoagulable disorders, systemic inflammatory conditions, hyperviscosity, malignancy, local infection, head trauma, and dural fistula.

Headache is the hallmark feature of CVST, present in 85% of patients, and in some patients it may be the only presenting symptom. The character of the headache varies, and onset is most typically gradual. Additional clinical features include seizures, focal signs, papilledema, and altered level of alertness or coma. Seizures are typically focal onset. Venous occlusion may cause edema, infarction, and/or ICH. As with other systemic venous thromboses, pulmonary embolism is a potentially fatal complication.

Diagnosis requires a high index of suspicion because symptoms may be nonspecific, and noncontrast head CT results may be normal. MRI is more sensitive for detecting cerebral ischemia or edema. Vascular imaging with magnetic resonance venography or CT venography are sensitive for the diagnosis; conventional angiography is rarely indicated. After establishing the diagnosis of CVST one should determine the etiology of the thrombosis. Evaluation for hypercoagulable states including protein C, protein S, and antithrombin deficiency; antiphospholipid syndrome; prothrombin G20210 mutation; and Factor V Leiden is appropriate in select patients. Additional workup should investigatefor these associated inciting factors. Of note, a substantial minority of patients have no clear inciting factor despite adequate evaluation.

Treatment consists of systemic anticoagulation with unfractionated or low-molecular weight heparin. It is of particular note that anticoagulation should be administered even in the presence of ICH. Heparin can be transitioned to a vitamin K antagonist for 3 to 12 months or indefinitely, depending on the etiology. In patients who are deteriorating clinically, mechanical clot disruption or catheter-directed thrombolysis are appropriate, although evidence for such treatment is limited. When local infections are present, antibiotics should be administered and/or surgical drainage should be done. Anticonvulsants are appropriate for patients in whom seizures occur, but are not indicated for prophylaxis. Patients with increased intracranial pressure should be monitored for vision loss and may be treated with acetazolamide, lumbar puncture, or ventricular shunting.

Recovery is often quite good in CVST, with 79% of patients having complete recovery at follow-up. However, the clinical course is variable and, without appropriate treatment, it may be fatal. As with many neurological conditions, appropriate treatment and prognostication must be customized to the particular patient's circumstances.

· CVST requires a high index of suspicion, particularly in patients with concerning headache features and thrombotic risk factors.

· Neuroimaging, including CT venography or magnetic resonance venography, is necessary when CVST is indicated clinically.

· Systemic anticoagulation is the treatment of choice, even in the presence of ICH.

Further Reading

Caplan LR. Cerebral venous thrombosis. In: *Caplan's Stroke: A Clinical Approach.* 4th ed. Philadelphia: Saunders/Elsevier; 2009:554–577.

Ferro JM, Canhão P, Stam J, et al. Prognosis of cerebral vein and dural sinus thrombosis: results of the International Study on Cerebral Vein and Dural Sinus Thrombosis (ISCVT). *Stroke.* 2004:35:664–670.

Piazza G. Cerebral venous thrombosis. *Circulation.* 2012;125:1704–1709.

Saposnik G, Barinagarrementeria F, Brown RD, et al. Diagnosis and management of cerebral venous thrombosis. *Stroke.* 2011;42:1158–1192.

Stam J. Thrombosis of the cerebral veins and sinuses. *N Engl J Med.* 2005;352:1791–1798.

3 Why Are You Staring over There?

Merritt W. Brown

A 45-year-old right-handed woman presents
with sudden onset of confusion and right
hemibody weakness that began 5 hours earlier.
On arrival at the emergency department she
is responsive and denies any impairment, but
her fluency is decreased. She raises her left
leg and arm when asked to raise her right,
and she does not respond to examiners or to
stimuli from the right side of her bed. Her gaze
deviates to the left. Her blood pressure is 143/
87, and her heart rate is 76 and regular. As time
progresses, she becomes more lethargic—to
the point at which she is intubated 8 hours
after her presentation because of profound
obtundation. On reexamination, her left pupil
has become dilated and is very sluggishly
reactive to light. She does not open her eyes
to noxious stimuli and is without very subtle

motor response to noxious stimuli on the left side, and a stereotyped, extensor posturing response is noted on her right side. The patient's blood pressure at this time is 193/98, and her heart rate is 51 and regular.

Her only history is a deep vein thrombosis. She is not on any anticoagulation medication, and her only medication is an oral contraceptive agent.

What do you do now?

MALIGNANT MIDDLE CEREBRAL ARTERY INFARCT

Discussion Questions

1. Based on her presentation, what is the most likely cause of her symptoms?
2. What could be causing her rapid decline?
3. What are the important symptoms to observe that would prompt expeditious action?
4. What interventions would you use to improve her likelihood of good outcome?

Discussion

This patient has several symptoms consistent with ischemia in the left middle cerebral artery (MCA) and possibly the anterior cerebral artery territory. Her right hemibody weakness results from ischemia and disruption of the primary motor cortex and axons from the left precentral gyrus. Her left gaze deviation with inability to cross the midline to the left can be explained by ischemia of the left frontal eye field resulting in unopposed action of the undamaged right frontal eye fields pushing gaze to the left, or by interruption of these fibers within the white matter projections from this region. The neglect of the right side of the patient's world most likely results from the disruption of the left frontal or parietal lobes, which encode for the spatial perception of the right side of the patient's world. Although spatial neglect is much better known as a result of nondominant parietal lobe damage, it can be seen in dominant (in our case, left) hemisphere damage as well. All these findings together strongly suggest a proximal left MCA or a distal intracranial internal cerebral artery lesion resulting in damage to a large territory of the left frontal and parietal lobes, or a hemorrhage that expands within these regions.

CT reveals a large, hypodense area within the left MCA territory suggestive of an ischemic infarct (Figure 3.1a).

Although she is rather young for such an event, her past history reveals multiple salient causes for her stroke, including oral contraceptive use as well as a history of hypercoagulability with regard to her deep vein thrombosis, possibly heralding some inborn procoaguable state not yet diagnosed.

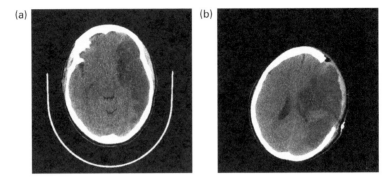

FIGURE 3.1 (a) Noncontrast head CT shows a large, hypodense area within the left middle cerebral artery (MCA) territory. (b) Large, left MCA infarct with cerebral edema and visible hemicraniectomy site with a calvarial deficit.

The concerning, precipitous decline of the patient is occurring most likely from herniation of the infarcted, edematous tissue downward against the brainstem, resulting in compression of the reticular activating system necessary for arousal and awake state Aside from her progressive obtundation, the acute mydriasis, or pupillary dilation, of her left eye serves as another clue to herniation. This finding most likely occurs from disruption of the parasympathetic fibers traveling on the superficial aspect of the oculomotor nerve. Unilateral mydriasis is a crucial indicator of herniation in patients with large-territory stroke or lesions causing mass effect and as such should prompt immediate action. Of note, younger patients in general are at a greater risk for these phenomena because of the relative volume of brain tissue compared with the more atrophied brains of stroke patients in later decades of life.

Treatment should be directed at the immediate relief of pressure against the brainstem. Neurosurgical intervention with hemicraniectomy, or removal of a portion of the skull, allows for swollen tissue to expand through the calvarial defect, relieving downward pressure against the brainstem (Figure 3.1b). Medically, hyperosmolar therapies such as hypertonic saline or mannitol allow for the elevation of intravascular oncotic pressure, thus decreasing the third-spacing of water from blood vessels into the infarcted tissue. Interventions such as hyperventilating a patient (usually by increasing the frequency of mechanical ventilation) can also reduce intracranial pressure by reducing intravascular carbon dioxide, a vasodilator, resulting in cerebral vasoconstriction, and thus decreasing the cerebral perfusion. The benefit of hyperventilation is only transient and should not be considered as long-term management for these patients. Rather, it is a temporizing intervention until more definitive therapy, such as hemicraniectomy, can be conducted. Also, raising the head of the bed 30° above the horizontal can help modestly in reducing cerebral perfusion pressure simply by exploiting gravity's effect of upward-traveling blood flow.

Expeditious use of such interventions in patients demonstrating signs of increasing intracranial pressure from edematous changes in infarcted tissue can prevent mortality; however, the underlying causal, large-territory infarct leaves the patient with considerable motor and perception deficits. As such, conversations with the patient's healthcare proxy, family, or other representatives are key to ensuring any interventions are congruent with the patient's beliefs and wishes.

KEY POINTS TO REMEMBER

- Patients with large-territory MCA infarcts should be monitored closely in a neurocritical care unit because they can develop significant, life-threatening cerebral edema.
- Medical management with hyperosmolar therapy, hyperventilation, and other measures should be done expeditiously if there are signs of increased intracranial pressure.
- Surgical management with hemicraniectomy should be offered, taking into account that it leads to increased survival at the cost of significant residual disability.
- The patient's age and prior wishes should be taken into account and discussed in detail with surrogate decision makers.

Further Reading

Holloway RG, Arnold RM, Creutzfeldt CJ, et al. Palliative and end-of-life care in stroke: a statement for healthcare professionals from the American Heart Association/American Stroke Association. *Stroke*. 2014;45(6):1887–1891.

Jüttler E, Unterberg A, Woitzik J, et al. Hemicraniectomy in older patients with extensive middle-cerebral-artery stroke. *N Engl J Med*. 2014;370(12):1091–1100.

Lukovits TG, Bernat JL. Ethical approach to surrogate consent for hemicraniectomy in older patients with extensive middle cerebral artery stroke. *Stroke*. 2014;45(9):2833–2835.

Vahedi K, Hofmeijer J, Juettler E, et al. Early decompressive surgery in malignant infarction of the middle cerebral artery: a pooled analysis of three randomised controlled trials. *Lancet Neurol*. 2007;6(3):215–222.

Wijdicks EF, Sheth KN, Carter BS, et al. Recommendations for the management of cerebral and cerebellar infarction with swelling: a statement for healthcare professionals from the American Heart Association/American Stroke Association. *Stroke*. 2014;45(4):1222–1238.

4 Dizziness and Ataxia after Lifting a Vacuum

Marc Bouffard

A 52-year-old woman presents to the emergency department with more than 24 hours of vertigo and nausea. She describes sudden-onset, room-spinning vertigo while lifting a heavy vacuum cleaner the day before presentation. The dizziness has been steady since then and does not improve with visual fixation. She can walk only with difficulty, and she falls to the left. There is neither tinnitus nor deafness. She denies any preceding illnesses.

Her past medical history includes hypertension, for which she takes lisinopril 10 mg daily. She is a life-long non-smoker and never uses drugs.

In the emergency department, her blood pressure is 181/81 and she has a heart rate of 60. She has mild left-sided ptosis. The left eye is hypotropic. The left pupil is 2 mm smaller than the right; the difference is accentuated in the dark. There is right-beating and counterclockwise nystagmus on right gaze, which does not extinguish. Saccades are hypermetric to the left and hypometric to the right. Her left face has diminished pinprick sensation. Left palatal activation is diminished. Pin and temperature sensation are diminished over the right hemibody. The left hand has a slight intention tremor and is dysmetric. On standing, her base is wide and she falls to the left if unsupported. She cannot walk without aid.

What do you do now?

LEFT LATERAL MEDULLARY SYNDROME CAUSED BY NONTRAUMATIC VERTEBRAL DISSECTION

Discussion Questions

1. Which areas of the nervous system have been affected?
2. What is the most likely vascular lesion and its cause?
3. How should you counsel the patient regarding treatment?

Discussion

There are several key clinical features in this patient that suggest lateral medullary pathology. Wallenberg's original description of his syndrome entailed vertigo, ipsilateral ataxia, and contralateral corporal hypoesthesia to pinprick and temperature. However, the original patient described by Wallenberg had preexisting pupillary abnormalities, and the association with Horner's syndrome was not recognized until later. The fact that pinprick sensation on the ipsilateral face is affected in the setting of preserved two-point discrimination implicates the spinal trigeminal tract, with sparing of the main nucleus of the trigeminal nerve in the pons. The spinal trigeminal tract descends as caudally as the upper cervical spine before decussation and ascension to the contralateral thalamus. The lack of ipsilateral palatal elevation is referable to the nucleus ambiguus, from which the somatic motor fibers of the glossopharyngeal nerve (CN IX) originate.

In addition, more subtle lateral medullary strokes may be diagnosed by recognizing often-overlooked neuro-ophthalmologic findings, which may be of diagnostic utility when the more widely known components of the lateral medullary syndrome are subtle or absent. Other findings that suggest lateral medullary pathology include lateropulsion and saccadic ataxia. The eyes may rest ipsilateral to the lesion rather than in the previous primary position. Saccades to the side of the lesion are hypermetric; saccades opposite the lesion are hypometric. Increasing the distance between the former and new targets of fixation accentuates the error. This is likely a process mediated by disruption of olivocerebellar fibers, resulting in poor motor control and possibly visuospatial function as well.

Laboratory testing showed a low-density lipoprotein level of 63 mg/dl, and hemoglobin A1c of 5.3%. Magnetic resonance angiography showed near occlusion of the left vertebral artery with a focal dissection. MRI showed a left posterolateral medullary infarct (Figure 4.1a).

The patient's lateral medullary stroke was the result of an occlusive dissection of the left vertebral artery (Figure 4.2). Radiographically, dissection may manifest as tapering of a vessel, resulting in stenosis or occlusion. Dissecting aneurysms are sometimes seen as well. On axial images, a flap associated with a false lumen and vascular narrowing may

(a)

(b)

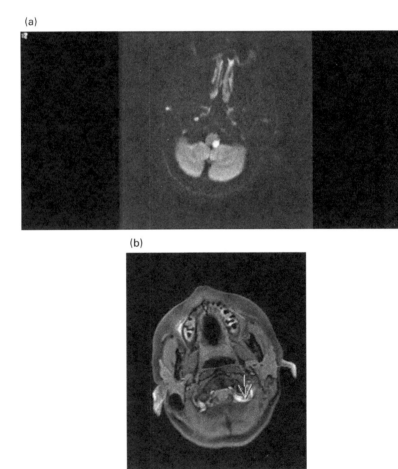

FIGURE 4.1 (a) Diffusion-weighted MRI with acute infarct in the last posterolateral medulla. (b) MRI with fat-saturated images highlighting the stenosed left vertebral artery with the mural hematoma (high-intensity signal).

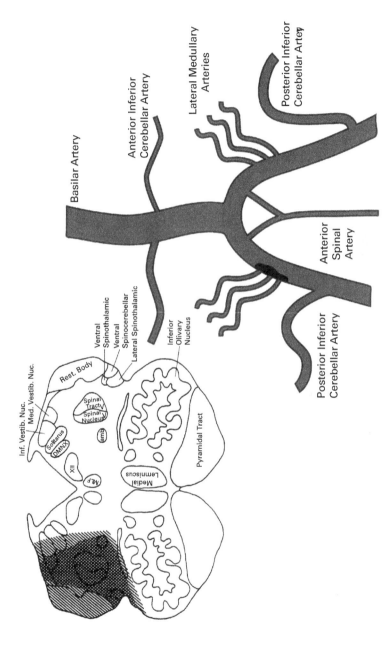

FIGURE 4.2 On the right is an artist's drawing of the occlusive vascular lesion within the intracranial vertebral artery that blocks flow in the arterial branches that supply the lateral medullary tegmentum. The figure in the upper left is the medulla, with the infarct shown by dark hatching.

be seen. The most sensitive means of imaging is T1-weighted MRI, with fat saturation sequences as a means of accentuating a mural hematoma (Figure 4.1b). The major radiographic differential diagnoses include complex and sometimes ruptured atheromas, dolichoectatic vessels, and fenestrated vessels.

There are several acknowledged risk factors for nontraumatic cervical artery dissection, although some have been studied more rigorously than others. Connective tissue diseases, including fibromuscular dysplasia, Ehlers-Danlos syndrome, Marfan's syndrome, and osteogenesis imperfecta (among others), have all been implicated. Although less than 2% of dissections are found to have one of the associated monogenic connective tissue disorders mentioned here, 50% of patients have structural connective tissue abnormalities manifest on skin biopsy that may be transmitted in an autosomal dominant manner. Inflammatory states such as recent infection, hyperhomocysteinemia, and autoimmune conditions (such as sarcoidosis) may be causes as well. Migraine and oral contraceptive use may be risk factors, but the mechanism in these cases is nebulous.

In general, recurrent stroke is uncommon after cervical artery dissection. The most recent data available suggest a risk of approximately 4% over 3 months following the initial dissection, although previous series suggested a greater risk. Theoretically, anticoagulants would be more effective in preventing propagation and embolization of the red clot that enters the lumen during a dissection. There are no studies that pit anticoagulants against antiplatelets during the first few days after dissection, which is, overwhelmingly, the most common time for recurrent stroke. There does not appear to be any significant difference between antiplatelet and anticoagulant therapy in terms of risk reduction for recurrent stroke or transient ischemic attack when treatment is begun after the first week. However, optimal management of cervical artery dissection on a case-by-case basis was heterogenous in the Antiplatelet treatment Compared with Anticoagulation Treatment for Cervical Artery Dissection (CADISS) trial and sometimes remains controversial when a multitude of individual patient factors are taken into account. Factors such as the etiology of dissection, length of dissection, and single versus multiple dissections have not been well studied.

- Major symptoms and signs in lateral medullary stroke include vertigo, nausea, ipsilateral ataxia, and Horner's syndrome.
- Subtle oculomotor abnormalities beyond nystagmus, such as saccadic ataxia, can have additional diagnostic and localization value.
- Arterial dissection can be the result of nontraumatic etiology and should always be considered in young patients with ischemic stroke.
- Optimal management to prevent stroke resulting from cervical artery dissections is not entirely clear. Antiplatelet agents and anticoagulation with warfarin seem equally effective. The decision is often made on a case-by-case basis.

Further Reading

Debette S, Leys D. Cervical-artery dissections: predisposing factors, diagnosis, and outcome. *Lancet Neurol.* 2009;8:668–678.

Khan SR, Lueck CJ. Hemi-seesaw nystagmus in lateral medullary syndrome. *Neurology.* 2013;80:1261–1262.

Morrow MM, Sharpe JA. Torsional nystagmus in the lateral medullary syndrome. *Ann Neurol.* 1988;24:390–398.

The CADISS trial investigators. Antiplatelet treatment compared with anticoagulation treatment for cervical artery dissection (CADISS): a randomized trial. *Lancet Neurol.* 2015;14:361–367.

Tilikete C, Koene A, Nighoghossian N, Vigetto A, Pelisson, D. Saccadic lateropulsion in Wallenberg syndrome: a window into cerebellar control of saccades? *Exp Brain Res.* 2006;174: 555–565.

Wallenberg A. Acute disease of the medulla. *Arch Psychiatrie.* 1985;24:509–540.

Yousem DM, Grossman RI. *Neuroradiology: The Requisites.* 3rd ed. Philadelphia: Mosby; 2010.

5 Two Generations with Stroke and Cognitive Decline

Shruti Sonni

A 62-year-old right-handed Hispanic man with a history of chronic headache, two recent ischemic strokes, and a recently resected left parietal meningioma presents with acute onset of left face, arm, and leg weakness. His blood pressure is 135/77. Key abnormal findings on examination are left hemiparesis with dysarthria and incoordination. In addition, the patient makes naming errors and has difficulty following complex commands. His medication list review shows he is taking atorvastatin and has been on warfarin since failing a regimen of aspirin and clopidogrel.

Review of his recent hospitalizations shows an extensive, unrevealing workup with transesophageal echocardiogram; CT scan of the chest, abdomen, and pelvis for occult malignancy; CT angiograms of the neck and head; lumbar puncture; hypercoagulability panel;

and a 30-day continuous heart monitor. His low-density lipoprotein is 69 mg/dL, his glycosylated hemoglobin is 5.7%, and his international normalized ratio is 2.3. The patient's family is especially concerned for his cognition, which has been declining steadily for the past several years. They mention the patient's father died at 55 years of age with dementia and "many small strokes."

What do you do now?

CADASIL

Discussion Questions

1. What are the possible anatomic localizations of the patient's neurological deficit?
2. What is the differential diagnosis?
3. How would you work up a patient with multiple infarcts of different ages?
4. How would you counsel the patient and family?

Discussion

Certain features of the clinical presentation offer hints that allow for a neuroanatomic localization and, consequently, generation of hypotheses regarding the underlying etiology, even before neuroimaging is obtained. Involvement of the arm, leg, and face in an equal degree is a key feature; it suggests a subcortical location with involvement of the white matter tract with high density of nerve fibers in close proximity with one another, such as the contralateral internal capsule or the base of the pons. Alternatively, an extensive hemisphere infarct involving the vast majority of the motor cortex could produce a similar motor deficit. However, such an extensive hemispheric infarct would inevitably result in other cortical deficits, such as neglect, cortical sensory loss, and visual field defect—all of which are lacking in this case. The patient's MRI confirms an acute infarct in the posterior limb of the right internal capsule (Figure 5.1a). The anomia and difficulty following commands might be the result of residual deficits from prior strokes, meningioma resection, or part of a parallel underlying process.

Lacunar infarcts are usually seen in the context of poorly controlled cardiovascular risk factors, especially hypertension and diabetes mellitus, both of which are lacking in this patient. Despite a very thorough and comprehensive workup, the stroke etiology has remained elusive, without atherosclerosis or other large-vessel vasculopathy, cardioembolic source, or a primary or secondary hypercoagulable state. The patient has had recurrent strokes despite dual antiplatelet coverage in the past, and therapeutic anticoagulation most recently. Alternative explanations should be pursued; most of the answers lie within the patient's history. His chronic headaches

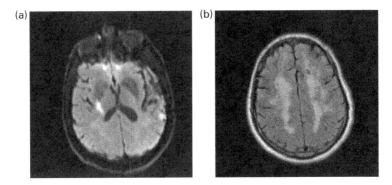

FIGURE 5.1 (a) Diffusion-weighted MRI showing acute infarct in the right internal capsule area. (b) Fluid-attenuated inversion recovery (FLAIR) MRI with extensive subcortical white matter hyperintensities.

are described as migraines with aura and they started during the last years of his third decade of life. Detailed collateral history from family members and careful cognitive examination reveal the extent of the patient's cognitive impairment is substantially worse than initially perceived. It also seems the patient's father had a very similar illness, with severe headaches, dementia, and recurrent small-vessel strokes. Last, his MRI shows very extensive, diffuse white matter lesions (Figure 5.1b), which are difficult to explain in the absence of vascular risk factors or a neuroinflammatory disorder or malignancy. These features, in light of an unrevealing thorough workup, raise concern for Cerebral Autosomal Dominant Arteriopathy with Subcortical Infarcts and Leukoencephalopathy, better known by the acronym *CADASIL*.

CADASIL is a small-vessel arteriopathy. Patients present with ischemic stroke, cognitive decline, migraine with aura (30% of cases) or psychiatric disturbances, "CADASIL coma" (an acute reversible encephalopathy), seizures, intracerebral hemorrhage, and, rarely, spinal infarcts. Migraine headaches occur early and seem to decrease after the first stroke. Multiple ischemic strokes and transient ischemic attacks occur in about 85% of cases, with a median age for ischemic stroke onset of approximately 50 years. The strokes present as a subcortical lacunar syndrome, although sometimes large-artery strokes have been reported. Strokes are recurrent, leading to severe disability with gait disturbance, urinary incontinence, and pseudobulbar palsy. Median age of severe disability is 64 years; median age of death is 68 years. Definitive diagnosis is confirmed with genetic testing, detecting mutations in the *NOTCH3* gene. Genetic screening does not detect all patients; skin biopsy, which is more specific, should be pursued if genetic testing is negative. This patient tested positive for the *NOTCH3* mutation. There is no targeted treatment for CADASIL, and management remains supportive. Angiography, anticoagulant therapy, and intravenous thrombolysis should be avoided because the risk of complications, mostly hemorrhagic, is high.

CADASIL is inherited in an autosomal dominant transmission pattern, which means each child of an affected patient has a 50% risk of inheriting the pathogenic variant. De novo mutations are rare and most patients have an affected parent. Asymptomatic, adult, first-degree relatives should receive genetic counseling before and after brain MRI, which might detect subclinical signs of CADASIL. Genetic testing for asymptomatic children is not recommended.

KEY POINTS TO REMEMBER

- Recurrent subcortical infarcts and cognitive decline in a patient with a history of complex migraine should raise concern for CADASIL, especially if there is family history.
- The condition is inherited in an autosomal dominant pattern with high penetrance, which means the children of an affected person have a 50% risk of inheriting the pathogenic gene.
- Screening asymptomatic children is not recommended.
- Anticoagulation and thrombolysis in the case of acute stroke should be avoided given the high risk for hemorrhagic complications.
- There is no effective treatment for CADASIL.

Further Reading

Caplan LR, Arenillas J, Cramer SC, et al. Stroke-related translational research. *Arch Neurol*. 2011;68(9):1110–1123.

Chabriat H, Bousser M-G. Cerebral Autosomal Dominant Arteriopathy with Subcortical Infarcts and Leukoencephalopathy (CADASIL). In: Caplan LR, ed. *Uncommon Causes of Stroke*. 2nd ed. Cambridge: Cambridge University Press; 2008:115–122.

Chabriat H, Joutel A, Dichgans M, et al. CADASIL. *Lancet Neurol*. 2009;8:643–653.

Chabriat H, Levy C, Taillia H, et al. Patterns of MRI lesions in CADASIL. *Neurology*. 1998;51:452–457.

Dichgans M. Genetics of ischaemic stroke. *Lancet Neurol*. 2007;6(2):149–161.

Dichgans M, Mayer M, Uttner I, et al. The phenotypic spectrum of CADASIL: clinical findings in 102 cases. *Ann Neurol*. 1998;44:731–739.

Pantoni L. Cerebral small vessel disease: from pathogenesis and clinical characteristics to therapeutic challenges. *Lancet Neurol*. 2010;9(7):689–701.

6   Ms. H Heads to the Hospital

Meg Van Nostrand

Ms. H is an 85-year-old woman who presents
after several days of "tipping to the right"
and subsequent development of right-sided
weakness. Her symptoms started 3 days
before her admission, with slight difficulty
walking, veering to her right, and "bumping
into things" on her right side. The patient
denies any double-vision, weakness, sensory
changes, or dizziness at that time. When she
tried to rise the following day, she found she
had developed significant right arm and leg
weakness. The right side of her face "felt
funny" and "tight," and she was drooling
out of the right corner of her mouth. Speech
production or comprehension remained intact
throughout.

   On examination she is afebrile with a blood
pressure of 181/84 and a regular heart rate. Mental
status and language examination are normal.
Decreased blink-to-threat over the right visual

hemifield and a flattened right nasolabial fold are noted. She has significant weakness in the right upper extremity, which is more pronounced distally, with essentially no movement beyond the elbow. The right leg is also weak, although less profoundly, and follows an upper motor neuron pattern. Sensory examination shows hypesthesia over the right hemibody.

Ms. H has a history of paroxysmal atrial fibrillation, hypertension, and hyperlipidemia. Her medications include propafenone for rate control and atorvastatin. Because of a history of significant gastrointestinal bleeding, warfarin was relatively contraindicated and she is maintained on aspirin and clopidogrel.

What do you do now?

ANTERIOR CHOROIDAL ARTERY INFARCT

Discussion Questions

1. What are plausible localizations for Ms. H's infarct?
2. Does the time course of Ms. H's presentation suggest a specific etiology?
3. Does the location of Ms. H's infarct suggest an etiology?
4. What diagnostic tests would help clarify the etiology?
5. How would defining the etiology affect treatment choices?

Discussion

This patient has a clinical syndrome of hemiparesis, hemihypesthesia involving the entire right hemibody, and right homonymous hemianopsia. A first thought would be that these symptoms suggest a large, left-hemispheric lesion involving a large part of the left middle cerebral artery territory. However, it would be virtually impossible for such a process not to result in at least some minor language deficit. Therefore, an alternative explanation should be sought. The triad of hemiplegia, hemisensory loss, and homonymous hemianopsia is classic for an anterior choroidal artery (AChA) territory infarction, with hemiplegia being the most common presenting symptom. Hemiplegia is a result of involvement of the posterior limb of the internal capsule, hemisensory loss results from the involvement of the ventral posterolateral nucleus of the thalamus, and hemianopsia results from involvement of the lateral geniculate body or geniculocalcarine tract.

The AChA originates from the terminal internal carotid artery just distal to the origin of the posterior communicating artery in the majority of individuals; although rarely it can originate from the proximal middle cerebral artery. The AChA supplies the lower two-thirds of the posterior limb of the internal capsule, internal segment of the globus pallidus, uncus, amygdala, and anterior hippocampus. Distally, it anastomoses with the posterior choroidal artery. There is a considerable degree of variability in the anatomy and supply of the AChA, which contributes to the relatively wide array of clinical symptoms that may be present with its infarction.

An alternative explanation is a lenticulostriate infarct that affects the posterior limb of the internal capsule and lateral thalamus. This is possible, although it would not account for the visual field deficit.

The patient's MRI indeed revealed an acute infarct in the left AChA territory (Figure 6.1).

The stuttering course of Ms. H's deficits seems to suggest small-vessel disease. Indeed, the AChA is a relatively small-caliber vessel and is susceptible to in situ atherosclerotic disease. Case series of AChA territory infarcts report considerable variance in the prevalence of several etiologies (small-vessel disease and large-vessel atherothrombosis, and cardioembolic and cryptogenic etiologies) with no true consensus on the most common etiology.

If Ms. H's stroke is in a location more compatible with a lenticulostriate infarct, the likelihood of small-vessel disease becomes much greater. Interestingly, a stuttering course of neurological deterioration is frequently found in AChA infarcts and is associated with a poor prognosis.

Fasting lipids, glycosylated hemoglobin, and blood pressure monitoring help to clarify the burden of vascular risk factors that could predispose patients to small-vessel disease. Transthoracic echocardiogram, telemetry monitoring, and vascular imaging (including the carotids) aid in determining the presence or absence of possible embolic sources.

The discovery of a cardioembolic source such as nonvalvular atrial fibrillation necessitates treatment with anticoagulation, given an absence of contraindications. If small-vessel disease is more likely, daily aspirin

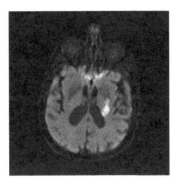

FIGURE 6.1 Diffusion-weighted MRI showing acute stroke in the left anterior choroidal artery territory.

administration and optimization of risk factors (lipids, glucose, and blood pressure) are the goals of treatment.

In this particular case, it is difficult to neglect the fact that the patient has a history of paroxysmal atrial fibrillation and, regardless of the factors mentioned earlier, which are mostly speculative considerations regarding the true nature of AChA infarcts, anticoagulation should be considered. Controlling the rest of her risk factors, such as blood pressure, hypercholesterolemia, and possible diabetes, is absolutely critical. The issue of anticoagulation is more complex. Combined aspirin and clopidogrel is not an optimal choice for cardioembolic stroke secondary prevention. Comorbidities, life expectancy, and the relative seriousness of complications should be taken into account. A gastrointestinal hemorrhage is a serious complication, but so is stroke, and the latter can have a profound effect on quality of life. In the absence of a documented lesion that predisposes her to gastrointestinal hemorrhage, treatment with warfarin with proper monitoring should not pose a significantly greater threat compared with aspirin/clopidogrel. Ultimately, the decision should be made with patient's input as well (although not left entirely to her!), ensuring she fully comprehends the risks and benefits.

KEY POINTS TO REMEMBER

- AChA infarcts result in a syndrome of hemiparesis, hemihypesthesia, and hemianopsia, without accompanying cortical signs expected in a large hemispheric infarct.
- The exact nature of the underlying stroke mechanism in AChA strokes is debatable; it is considered a small vessel by some and a large vessel by others.
- Regardless of the debate regarding the true underlying nature of the vessel, a full stroke workup should be pursued in cases of AChA stroke.

Further Reading

Bruno A, Graff-Radford NR, Biller J, Adams HP Jr. Anterior choroidal artery territory infarction: a small vessel disease. *Stroke*. 1989;20:616–619.

Chausson N, Joux J, Saint-Vil M et al. Infarction in the anterior choroidal artery territory: clinical progression and prognosis factors. *J Stroke Cerebrovasc Dis*. 2014;23(8):2012–2017.

Derflinger S, Fiebach JB, Böttger S, Haberl RL, Audebert HJ. The progressive course of neurological symptoms in anterior choroidal artery infarcts. *Int J Stroke*. 2015;10(1):134–137.

Helgason C, Caplan LR. Anterior choroidal artery-territory infarction: report of cases and review. *Arch Neurol*. 1986;43:681–686.

Leys D, Mounier-Vehier F, Lavenu I, Rondepierre P, Pruvo JP. Anterior choroidal artery territory infarcts: study of presumed mechanisms. *Stroke*. 1994;25:837–842.

Palomeras E, Fossas P, Cano AT, Sanz P, Floriach M Anterior choroidal artery infarction: a clinical, etiologic and prognostic study. *Acta Neurol Scand*. 2008;118:42-47.

Ropper MV, Allan H. *Adams and Victor's Principles of Neurology*. 7th ed. New York: McGraw-Hill; 2001.

7 The Weak Construction Worker

Mark McAllister

A 49-year-old right-handed construction worker presents to the emergency department because of right-sided numbness and weakness as well as headache. He was at work, carrying tools, when he noted tingling and numbness on his right side. Coworkers noted right-sided facial droop and slurred speech. Weakness of the left arm and leg followed, as did a holocephalic headache. He presents to the emergency department by ambulance 2 hours after symptom onset. He denies taking any medications and has not seen a doctor for more than 15 years, but admits to being told previously that he has "heart problems" and has been prescribed a "pressure pill" that he no longer takes.

His heart rate is 104 and regular, and his blood pressure is 204/116. Neurological examination is notable for normal alertness; moderate dysarthria; severe weakness of the right face, arm, and leg; and markedly decreased pinprick sensation on the right hemibody.

What do you do now?

HYPERTENSIVE PRIMARY INTRACEREBRAL HEMORRHAGE

Discussion Questions

1. What is the most likely diagnosis?
2. How should the patient be evaluated?

Discussion

Because this patient presents with sudden onset of progressive, lateralized deficits and headache, the etiology must be presumed vascular until proved otherwise. The differential diagnosis consists primarily of acute ischemic stroke (AIS) and intracerebral hemorrhage (ICH), with cerebral venous sinus thrombosis (CVST), seizure, migraine, and mass lesion being less likely. Emergent neuroimaging is indicated, and a noncontrast head CT showed a left thalamocapsular hemorrhage measuring 61 mm at its broadest, largest dimension (Figure 7.1).

Clinical features of ICH are similar to those of AIS, and neuroimaging is a necessity because they cannot be distinguished reliably. Both CT and MRI are sensitive for ICH, although CT may be available more rapidly. In addition to focal signs, headache, seizures, vomiting, and decreased alertness may be present. The most common locations of ICH are deep structures—basal ganglia, thalamus, pons, and cerebellum—followed by lobar hemorrhages.

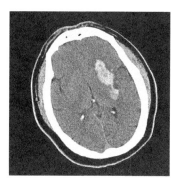

FIGURE 7.1 Noncontrast head CT reveals a hematoma in the left basal ganglia area, in close proximity to the internal capsule and the lateral thalamus.

Hypertension is the most common cause of ICH; both chronic and acute increases in blood pressure can precipitate hemorrhage. Other possible etiologies include disorders of coagulation (especially prescribed anticoagulants), cerebral amyloid angiopathy, trauma, drug and use (particularly cocaine and amphetamines); rarer causes include tumors, vascular malformations, CVST, reversible cerebral vasoconstriction syndrome, and vasculitis.

Based on the patient's history, reasonable investigations may include complete blood count, coagulation studies, toxicology screening, vascular imaging, and contrast-enhanced MRI. It is worth noting that novel oral anticoagulants do not necessarily cause abnormalities on routine coagulation studies. Evaluation with CT angiography may show evidence of an underlying arteriovenous malformation, but does not show cavernous angiomas because they lack feeding vessels. Extravasation of intravenous contrast into the hematoma, the so-called "spot sign," is predictive of hematomas that are likely to expand. MRI may show diffuse microbleeds characteristic of cerebral amyloid angiopathy or evidence of an underlying tumor, although blood products may obscure interpretation. Venography with CT or MRI should be performed when CVST is suspected.

Treatment depends on initial stabilization, including transfer to a critical care unit if necessary. Blood pressure should be treated aggressively to achieve a systolic blood pressure of less than 140 mm Hg, which may require the use of intravenous drips. If the patient has a bleeding diathesis or is anticoagulated, one should withhold anticoagulation and apply the appropriate reversal agent. For those taking vitamin K antagonists, fresh-frozen plasma and/or prothrombin complex concentrates should be administered in addition to vitamin K. There are no evidence-based strategies for reversal of novel oral anticoagulants. For patients with severe hemorrhages or clinical deterioration, surgical decompression and drainage may be considered, although the decision to proceed with surgery should be individualized in consultation with an experienced neurosurgeon.

Anticonvulsants should be administered in patients with seizures, but routine prophylaxis is not recommended. Fever and hyperglycemia are associated with worse outcomes in ICH and should be treated. Medical venous thromboembolism prophylaxis should be avoided initially but may be resumed 1 to 4 days after onset, when stabilization of the hematoma has been determined with repeat imaging.

For this patient, there were no abnormalities on his coagulation panel and toxicology screen. There was no evidence of an underlying vascular abnormality on CT angiography. The most likely etiology of his ICH is chronically untreated hypertension. After initial therapy, he needs to be placed on a chronic antihypertensive regimen and be referred to a rehabilitation facility.

The prognosis of ICH is variable and is related primarily to hemorrhage location and size. Mass effect and herniation are the greatest immediate threats to life. Preventing recurrence is focused on treating the underlying etiology of the ICH.

KEY POINTS TO REMEMBER

- ICH presents similarly to AIS, and rapid neuroimaging is critical to differentiate between the diagnoses.
- Hypertension is the most common cause of ICH, and early aggressive blood pressure management is critical to prevent hematoma expansion.
- There are numerous causes of ICH and the evaluation must be tailored to individual patient characteristics.

Further Reading

Caplan LR. Intracerebral hemorrhage. In: *Caplan's Stroke: A Clinical Approach.* 4th ed. Philadelphia: Saunders/Elsevier; 2009:487–522.

Hemphill JC, Greenberg SM, Anderson CS, et al. Guidelines for the management of spontaneous intracerebral hemorrhage. *Stroke.* 2015;46:2032–2060.

Nyquist P. Management of acute intracranial and intraventricular hemorrhage. *Crit Care Med.* 2010;38:946–953.

Qureshi AI, Mendelow AD, Hanley DF. Intracerebral haemorrhage. *Lancet.* 2009;373:1632–1644.

Tsivgoulis G, Katsanos AH, Butcher KS, et al. Intensive blood pressure reduction in acute intracerebral hemorrhage: a meta-analysis. *Neurology.* 2014;83:1523–1529.

8 Twisted Tongue and Dizzy Head

Bart Chwalisz and Elorm Avakame

A 36-year-old right-handed man with no prior medical history presents with a sudden onset of headache, vertigo, and right arm and leg weakness and numbness.

About a week before presentation, the patient experienced some violent coughing episodes in the setting of seasonal allergies, after which he noticed pain in the left side of his posterior neck. The morning of presentation, he twisted his head and neck while bending down to pick up his son, at which point he immediately experienced sudden onset of severe left neck pain and headache, and severe vertigo. After 30 minutes his vertigo improved somewhat. About 3 hours later, he developed dysarthria and right arm and leg numbness and weakness. The patient has no significant prior medical history, takes no medication, and denies use of tobacco products or illicit drugs.

On examination. his blood pressure is 127/89. He is awake and cooperative, but uncomfortable. Moderate dysarthria is noted. Visual fields are full. Pupils are equal without ptosis. Eye movements are intact, with nystagmus when looking to the right. Hearing, facial sensation, and strength are intact. The palate does not elevate on the left. His tongue deviates to the left. The motor examination shows significant variability. During the initial examination, he had antigravity strength in the right arm and leg but, when examined a few hours later while sitting up, he has become completely plegic in the right arm and leg.

Sensation is diminished to light touch (but intact to pinprick) on the right arm and leg. Coordination cannot be tested on the right, given the severity of weakness, but is intact on the left. He cannot ambulate.

What do you do now?

MEDIAL MEDULLARY INFARCT

Discussion Questions

1. Where would you localize the lesion?
2. What is the likely mechanism?
3. What is your next step in the diagnostic workup?
4. What is the management of this patient?

Discussion

Notable findings include a crossed pattern of deficits: impaired cranial nerves X (palate elevation) and XII (tongue control) on the left, with impaired sensation and strength on the right body below the neck. This immediately suggests a brainstem lesion. More specifically, the lower cranial nerve dysfunction puts the lesion in the medulla. The affected structures lie in the medullary midline: the hypoglossal nerve fascicles, medial lemniscus (dorsal column sensory modalities), and pyramids (corticospinal motor function). More lateral-lying structures (such as the spinothalamic tract, spinal nucleus and tract of V, descending sympathetics, and restiform body) are not affected.

The neuroanatomic diagnosis is medial medullary syndrome (also known as *Dejerine syndrome*).

The rapid onset of fixed neurological deficits suggests a stroke. The strictly lateralized deficits respect vascular boundaries. As mentioned, although the clinical deficits are extensive, they can all be explained by disruption of a small area in the left medial medulla—an area that falls in the territory of a direct perforating branch from the left vertebral artery. It is also notable that the development of the deficits was preceded by a discrete, transient vertiginous episode. Although not specific, vertigo is suggestive of a posterior circulation stroke or transient attack in the posterior circulation. Moreover, this symptom is not readily explained by medial medullary dysfunction. Thus, it can be surmised the patient experienced two independent events in quick succession, at two different locations, but both within the posterior circulation. This suggests embolization originating from the left vertebral artery or, less likely, a more proximal source, such as the heart or the aortic arch.

This young man has no prior medical history and no obvious stroke risk factors. He did, however, experience recent neck pain on the left, precipitated initially by severe cough, then—on the day of presentation—triggered by a sudden head movement. This history is concerning for a left vertebral dissection with distal embolization.

The suspicion of dissection is high and should be confirmed with vascular imaging. In the emergency room setting, CT angiography (CTA) of the neck and head would provide appropriately fast imaging of the area in question. Head CT is insensitive for small strokes in the posterior circulation, and it would likely not show the lesion. MRI could be done as a second step to confirm the presence of stroke. Magnetic resonance angiography (MRA) would also show the vascular lesion with similar sensitivity, but acquisition is slower.

CTA was done and was concerning for vertebral dissection, but it was not conclusive. MRA with fat-saturated images clearly demonstrated a dissection of the left vertebral artery (Figure 8.1a). MRI confirmed the presence of an anteromedial medullary stroke (Figure 8.1b).

During the acute phase, a suspected or demonstrated arterial dissection is not a contraindication to tissue plasminogen activator. An antithrombotic agent should be started to prevent further embolization. In a meta-analysis, anticoagulation with warfarin was not found to be superior with aspirin. It is also felt that the presence of intradural dissection is a relative contraindication to anticoagulation, because the vessel wall there has a

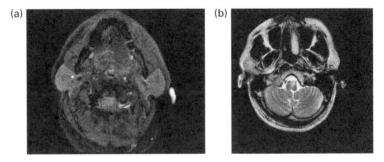

(a)   (b)

FIGURE 8.1 (a) Fat-saturated MRI showing mural hematoma and irregularity in the wall of the left vertebral artery (high-intensity signal). (b) T2 MRI sequence with acute left anteromedial medullary infarct.

thin media and adventitia, and fewer elastic fibers, and may be more prone to rupture.

One notable feature in this patient's examination is that the severity of the findings fluctuated. When examined a few hours after presentation, his motor examination had worsened significantly, and the examining neurologist noticed this occurred after the patient sat up. When the bed was lowered, the motor deficit became much milder. This confirmed there was a postural component to the patient's infarct. He was treated with intravenous fluids and maintained on flat bed rest for several days until perfusion improved and he ceased to have gravity-dependent motor fluctuations.

KEY POINTS TO REMEMBER

· Crossed deficits (cranial nerve involvement on one side, with contralateral long-tract signs such as weakness or sensory loss) suggest a brainstem localization.

· In the brainstem, strictly lateralized deficits suggest infarct as the etiology because they reflect involvement of specific vascular territories.

· Neck pain with lateralized neurological deficits suggests arterial dissection. One should also especially consider dissection as a stroke mechanism in young individuals, associated with trauma or unusual head positions (e.g., chiropractor, hairdresser), or in individuals with either a family history or physical features of a connective tissue disorder. However, remember that dissection can occur with trivial trauma or even with no recollection of trauma whatsoever!

· Diagnosis of dissection can be made with CTA, MRA, or conventional angiogram. In borderline cases, MRA with fat-saturated images can be diagnostic.

· Anticoagulation with warfarin has not been shown to be superior to aspirin and may increase the risk of subarachnoid hemorrhage if dissection is intradural.

· If a patient's stroke-related deficits seem to fluctuate, check whether they are gravity dependent! In some cases, optimizing perfusion by putting the head of the bed flat and administering fluids can improve neurological function quickly.

Further Reading

Kennedy F, Lanfranconi S, Hicks C, et al. Antiplatelets vs anticoagulation for dissection: CADISS nonrandomized arm and meta-analysis. *Neurology.* 2012; 79(7):686–689.

Kim JS, Han YS. Medial medullary infarction: clinical, imaging, and outcome study in 86 consecutive patients. *Stroke.* 2009;40:3221–3225.

Lee MJ, Park YG, Kim SJ, et al. Characteristics of stroke mechanisms in patients with medullary infarction. *Eur J Neurol.* 2012;19(11):1433–1439.

Provenzale JM. MRI and MRA for evaluation of dissection of craniocerebral arteries: lessons from the medical literature. *Emerg Radiol.* 2009; 16(3):185–193.

Provenzale JM, Sarikaya B. Comparison of test performance characteristics of MRI, MR angiography, and CT angiography in the diagnosis of carotid and vertebral artery dissection: a review of the medical literature. *AJR Am J Roentgenol* 2009;193(4):1167–1174.

9 Right Hemibody Weakness in a Man with Lightning-like Transient Facial Pain

D. Eric Searls

A 75-year-old man presents to the emergency department with 5 hours of right-sided hemiparesis and dysarthria. One week before presentation he had a transient episode of right face, arm, and leg weakness, and dysarthria that lasted 30 minutes with complete resolution. For about a year he had daily, brief, left-sided lancinating excruciating facial pains. The facial pain is triggered and exacerbated by chewing or touching the left side of his face.

The patient's past medical history is significant for hypertension, hyperlipidemia, and cigarette smoking (30 pack-years). His medications include hydrochlorothiazide 25 mg daily and atorvastatin 20 mg. On examination, his blood pressure is 160/92, and his pulse is 76 and regular. He is afebrile. No carotid or vertebral bruits are auscultated. Neurological examination is notable for moderate dysarthria, hypersensitivity to touch and pinprick in the left V2 region of his face, right lower facial droop, and severe weakness of the right arm and leg in an upper motor neuron distribution. A fasting lipid panel reveals a total cholesterol of 220 mg/dL and low-density lipoprotein of 160 mg/dL. Noncontrast brain CT does not show an infarct or hemorrhage.

What do you do now?

VERTEBROBASILAR DOLICHOECTASIA

Discussion Questions

1. What type of lesion is most likely and where is it localized?
2. What is the most probable causative mechanism?
3. What treatment would you recommend?

Discussion

The time course of this patient's presentation—in particular, the occurrence of a transient syndrome of right-sided hemiparesis followed a week later by persistent symptoms of the same type—strongly suggests a transient ischemic attack followed by a stroke. The symptoms of an intraparenchymal hemorrhage would be highly unlikely to resolve after 30 minutes, and would be unlikely to recur in the same distribution a week later. A complex partial seizure with postictal paresis is unlikely, given the patient did not report a change in mental status or tonic/clonic activity. Symptoms of a space-occupying lesion such as neoplasm would be highly unlikely to resolve in 30 minutes. Given this patient's age, a demyelinating disease would be highly improbable.

The occurrence of dysarthria and right-sided hemiparesis may localize to the pyramidal tracts of the left hemisphere or left brainstem. Because the patient's weakness appears to affect the face, arm, and leg relatively equally, this further suggests the lesion may be in the pons, the posterior limb of the internal capsule, or the basal ganglia. One clue is offered by the daily, brief episodes of lancinating pain on the left side of his face. These episodes suggest that he is having trigeminal neuralgia. Sometimes, trigeminal neuralgia is triggered by an artery compressing or irritating the trigeminal nerve as it leaves the pons.

Brain MRI showed an acute small infarct involving the left pontine base on diffusion-weighted imaging (Figure 9.1a). An ectatic basilar artery that deviated to the left and compressed the left trigeminal nerve can be seen in the T2 sequence of the brain MRI (Figure 9.1b). The patient has a dolichoectatic basilar artery with midbasilar atherosclerotic disease, demonstrated in his CT Angiogram (Figure 9.1c). The dolichoectatic vessel is also compressing the left trigeminal nerve, resulting in trigeminal neuralgia

Dolichoectasia refers to dilated and tortuous arteries, more often in the posterior circulation rather than in the anterior circulation. Dolichoectatic vessels can arise as a result of atherosclerosis, congenital causes, or dissection. Atherosclerotic dolichoectasia occurs most often in patients older than 40, especially men, and tends to affect the intracranial vertebral and basilar arteries. Congenital dolichoectasia typically affects patients younger than 40, especially woman. Diseases that may predispose to congenital dolichoectasia include Marfan's syndrome,

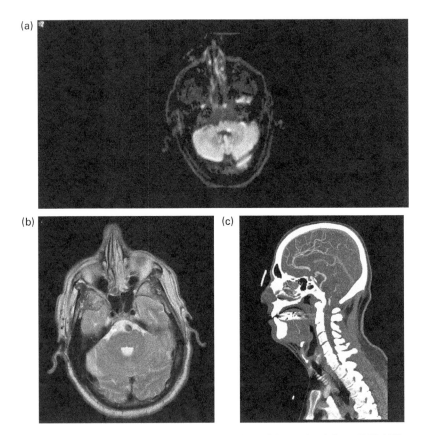

FIGURE 9.1 (a) Diffusion-weighted MRI with acute left medial medullary infarct. (b) T2 MRI sequence showing a tortuous and dilated basilar artery with intraluminal thrombus. Notice the indentation of the dilated vessel and focal pressure on the left side of the brainstem. (c) Sagittal view of CT angiogram with visualization of the tortuosity and luminal irregularity of the basilar artery.

Ehlers-Danlos syndrome, AIDS, Fabry's disease, sickle cell anemia, and alpha-glucosidase deficiency. Other vascular malformations bear similarities to dolichoectasia. Fusiform aneurysms are ectatic vessels with a focal aneurysmal outpouching. Large fusiform aneurysms are referred to as *giant serpentine aneurysms.*

Dolichoectasia can predispose to stroke via several mechanisms. Ectatic vessels often have abnormal blood flow with sharply decreased blood flow velocities. Flow can be turgid and can even reverse direction. Decreased blood flow can result in thrombus formation. Atherosclerotic plaques, sometimes with calcification, may protrude into the artery lumen and facilitate thrombus formation. Thrombi may block the lumen of branch arteries or embolize distally. Elongated and tortuous arteries may distort the orifices of branch arteries, especially in the pons, thereby decreasing flow and causing infarcts. Fragile dolichoectatic arteries may rupture and cause subarachnoid hemorrhage or intracranial hemorrhage.

Treatment of dolichoectasia remains uncertain. Antiplatelet or anticoagulant treatments have limited effectiveness, perhaps because of multiple stroke mechanisms other than atherosclerosis. Caution is advised in giving antiplatelets or anticoagulants to patients with vertebrobasilar dolichoectasia who present with symptoms other than ischemia (e.g., hemifacial spasm or cranial nerve deficits).

Whether to pursue surgical treatment of dolichoectatic arteries and fusiform aneurysms is often unclear, and the intervention itself can be challenging. Unlike saccular aneurysms, these vessels lack a definable neck that can be clipped surgically while still preserving the parent vessel. Surgical intervention may cause bleeding or may compromise the distal blood supply. Some surgical options include trapping with bypass, proximal occlusion, resection with anastomosis, and transposition.

KEY POINTS TO REMEMBER

- Dolichoectatic vessels may be atherosclerotic or congenital, or the result of dissections.
- Dolichoectasia may cause ischemic strokes, hemorrhagic strokes, cranial nerve deficits, brainstem compression, and hydrocephalus.

- Potential mechanisms for ischemic stroke include hemodynamic, intraluminal thrombus occluding the opening of brainstem branch arteries, artery-to-artery embolism, small-vessel ischemic disease, and dissection.
- The optimal noninvasive imaging techniques are CT angiography and magnetic resonance angiography with contrast. Conventional angiogram remains the gold standard.
- Prognosis is highly variable, ranging from asymptomatic or few deficits to severe deficits. Recurrent ischemia is much more likely than recurrent intracranial hemorrhage.
- The best treatment approach remains unclear. Antiplatelets or anticoagulation are often used. However, caution is recommended in giving antiplatelets or anticoagulation to patients who present with nonischemic symptoms (i.e., cranial nerve deficits).

Further Reading

Anson JA, Lawton MT, Spetzler RF. Characteristics and surgical treatment of dolichoectatic and fusiform aneurysms. *J Neurosurg*. 1996;84:185–193.

Flemming KD, Wiebers DO, Brown RD Jr, et al. The natural history of radiographically defined vertebrobasilar nonsaccular intracranial aneurysms. *Cerebrovasc Dis*. 2005;20:270–279.

Passero SG, Calchetti B, Bartalini S. Intracranial bleeding in patients with vertebrobasilar dolichoectasia. *Stroke*. 2005;36:1421–1425.

Passero SG, Rossi S. Natural history of vertebrobasilar dolichoectasia. *Neurology*. 2008;70:66–72.

Pico F, Labreuche J, Amarenco P. Pathophysiology, presentation, prognosis, and management of intracranial arterial dolichoectasia. *Lancet Neurol*. 2015;14: 833–845.

Pico F, Labreuche J, Touboul P-J, Leys D, Amarenco P. Intracranial arterial dolichoectasia and its relation with atherosclerosis and stroke subtype. *Neurology*. 2003;61:1736–1742.

Savitz S, Caplan LR. Dilatative arteriopathy (dolichoectasia). In Caplan LR, ed. *Uncommon Causes of Stroke*. 2nd ed. New York: Cambridge University Press; 2008:479–482.

Savitz S, Ronthal M, Caplan LR. Vertebral artery compression of the medulla. *Arch Neurol*. 2006;63:234–241.

10 Blurry Vision

D. Eric Searls

A 64-year-old man presents to the emergency
department with 20 minutes of a visual
disturbance in his right eye that developed
that morning as he was sitting. He describes
a "graying of my vision" that starts superiorly
in the right eye and descends over several
seconds to the horizontal meridian. He has
difficulty distinguishing details in his superior
field. He closes one eye at a time and confirms
that only the right eye is affected. After 20
minutes, the "gray curtain" lifts over several
seconds, starting inferiorly and progressing
superiorly. His vision returns to baseline.

His blood pressure is 148/88 and he has a regular
pulse of 84. He has a right carotid bruit and poor
dorsalis pedis pulses bilaterally. Ophthalmologic
examination shows bright, yellow-orange, round
plaques within retinal arteries in both eyes
without hemorrhages or papilledema. His visual
acuity is 20/30 in both eyes. Visual fields are

intact to confrontation bilaterally. Otherwise, his neurological examination is intact.

His past medical history includes hypertension, hyperlipidemia, type 2 diabetes, and peripheral vascular disease. He has never had a similar visual disturbance. Medications include amlodipine, atorvastatin, and metformin, but not an antiplatelet agent.

What do you do now?

TRANSIENT MONOCULAR VISUAL LOSS RESULTING FROM CAROTID STENOSIS

Discussion Questions

1. What does the patient's clinical presentation suggest and what are its possible etiologies?
2. What type of laboratory and imaging workup is indicated?
3. How would you treat this patient?

Discussion

This patient's symptoms can be described as transient monocular visual loss (TMVL). Several different terms, including *amaurosis fugax* and *transient monocular blindness*, have been used to describe TMVL in the literature, thereby causing confusion. Patient vagueness in symptom description adds to the diagnostic confusion. "Blurry vision" is very often all the clinician will get from the patient, and very few patients attempt to distinguish between monocular and binocular symptoms. Luckily, this patient was particularly accurate and his symptom description, leading to more directed hypotheses regarding the underlying process.

Many vascular and ophthalmologic etiologies can produce TMVL; however, the described visual deficit and the pattern of involvement strongly suggest a vascular etiology. Embolism from the internal carotid artery to the eye's arterial supply is a frequent vascular etiology (Figure 10.1). This can occur as a result of atheromatous disease or dissection. There is no reason to suspect dissection in a patient of this age without recent head or neck injury, headache, or neck pain. Cardiac or aortic arch embolism happens, but less frequently. Hypoperfusion, retinal artery venous occlusion, and retinal migraine are other potential vascular causes, but the clinical examination and presentation do not suggest any of these. Temporal arteritis and nonarteritic anterior ischemic optic neuropathy more frequently produce persistent rather than transient vision loss. Other nonvascular optic neuropathies are possible but less likely. Optic neuritis is typically associated with eye pain and loss of color vision. Acute intermittent glaucoma, colobomas, and optic disc drusen may cause TMVL and it is prudent to exclude by an ophthalmology consultation.

Fundoscopy is essential. The appearance of possible embolic particles within retinal arteries can give clues regarding the type and origin of emboli. The presence of unilateral papilledema suggests an acute event resulting from inflammation or ischemia. Optic disc pallor is more likely a subacute or chronic event, occurring at 4 to 6 weeks. Visual acuity and visual fields must also be assessed.

For patients older than 50 years erythrocyte sedimentation rate and C-reactive protein should be checked to exclude temporal arteritis, especially if there is headache or systemic symptoms. If these levels are elevated, or if the presentation is concerning for temporal arteritis, then steroids should be started and a temporal artery biopsy obtained. Initiation of steroids should not be delayed until the biopsy results are known, because treatment delay may lead to permanent vision loss. Patients with TMVL who are older than 50, or younger patients with multiple vascular risk factors, should undergo brain and vascular imaging. Vascular imaging could include magnetic resonance angiography of the brain and neck, CT angiography of the brain and neck, or carotid ultrasound. If no carotid stenosis is found, then a transthoracic echocardiogram should be obtained. Patients who are suspected to be hypercoagulable should have a hypercoagulability panel checked.

Laboratory testing for this patient showed an erythrocyte sedimentation rate of 20 mm/hr and C-reactive protein of 0.5 mg/L. The fasting lipid panel indicated a low-density lipoprotein level of 190 mg/dl, total cholesterol of 320 mg/dl, and high-density lipoprotein of 30 mg/dl. Transthoracic echocardiogram did not show a cardiac clot or aortic arch atheroma. Telemetry did not reveal an arrhythmia. Brain MRI showed no infarct. Brain and neck magnetic resonance angiography were remarkable for 40% to 50% stenosis of the right proximal internal carotid artery.

In the absence of other explanatory diagnoses, this patient's symptoms are very likely the result of an embolus from a mildly stenosed right proximal internal carotid artery to an inferior retinal artery of the right eye.

This patient should be treated with an antiplatelet medication and his statin dose should be increased. Because he has only mild stenosis of his right proximal internal carotid artery, he is not a candidate for a carotid endarterectomy or stenting procedure. Those patients with TMVL resulting from embolism from moderate (50%–69%) or severe (70%–99%)

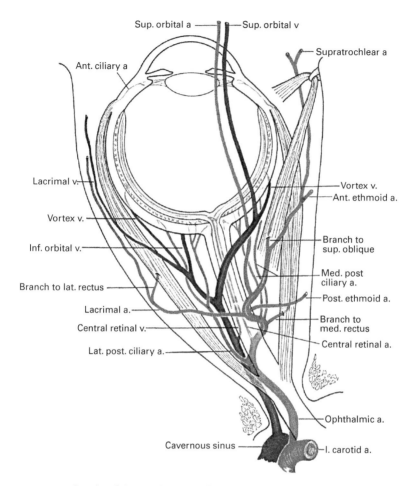

Sup. orbital a —— ——Sup. orbital v

Supratrochlear a

Ant. ciliary a

Lacrimal v.

Vortex v.

Inf. orbital v.

Branch to lat. rectus

Lacrimal a.

Central retinal v.

Lat. post. ciliary a.

Vortex v.
Ant. ethmoid a.

Branch to
sup. oblique

Med. post
ciliary a.

Post. ethmoid a.

Branch to
med. rectus

Central retinal a.

Ophthalmic a.

Cavernous sinus

I. carotid a.

FIGURE 10.1   Drawing of the vascular supply of the eye.

Source: From Caplan LR (ed) (1995), Brain Ischemia: Basic Concepts and Clinical Relevance, London, Springer-Verlag, with permission.

carotid stenosis—and especially those with ulcerated or hemorrhagic plaques—should be considered for carotid endarterectomy or stenting.

KEY POINTS TO REMEMBER

· TMVL may be the result of thromboembolic disease, temporal arteritis, nonarteritic anterior ischemic optic neuropathy, retinal migraine, other vascular causes (dissection, vasculitis, vascular malformations), and ocular causes.

- TMVL occurs more frequently as a result of emboli from the proximal internal carotid artery than from the heart or aorta.
- Patients who have an initial episode of TMVL as a result of a thromboembolic mechanism have half the risk of subsequent hemispheric stroke compared with patients who present initially with hemispheric stroke.
- Thorough physical, ophthalmologic, and neurological examinations are essential for discovering the etiology of TMVL. Retinal findings may suggest the origin of retinal emboli.
- Temporal arteritis is a preventable cause of permanent visual loss. If there is clinical suspicion for temporal arteritis, treatment with steroids must begin immediately.
- Patients with TMVL who are older than 50 years, or younger patients with multiple vascular risk factors, should undergo magnetic resonance brain and vascular imaging.

Further Reading

Benavente O, Eliasziw M, Streifler JY, et al. Prognosis after transient monocular blindness associated with carotid-artery stenosis. *N Engl J Med.* 2001;345:1084–90.

Bruno A, Corbett JJ, Biller J, et al. Transient monocular visual loss patterns and associated vascular abnormalities. *Stroke.* 1990;21:34.

Caselli RJ, Hunder GG, Whisnant JP. Neurologic disease in biopsy-proven giant cell (temporal) arteritis. *Neurology.* 1988;38:352–359.

Donders RC. Clinical features of transient monocular blindness and the likelihood of atherosclerotic lesions of the internal carotid artery. *J Neurol Neurosurg Psychiatry.* 2001;71:247.

Fisher CM. Transient monocular blindness versus amaurosis fugax. *Neurology.* 1989;39:1622–1624.

Hayreh SS, Zimmerman MB. Incipient nonarteritic anterior ischemic optic neuropathy. *Ophthalmology.* 2007;114:1763–1772.

North American Symptomatic Carotid Endarterectomy Trial collaborators. Beneficial effect of carotid endarterectomy in symptomatic patients with high-grade stenosis. *N Engl J Med.* 1991;325:445–453.

Pessin MS, Duncan GW, Mohr JP, Poskanzer DC. Clinical and angiographic features of carotid transient ischemic attacks. *N Engl J Med.* 1977;296:358.

11 Gastroenteritis with Dizziness and Ataxia

Lester Y. Leung

A 38-year-old man had 2 days of dizziness, nausea,
vomiting, diarrhea, and reduced intake of food and
fluids. He awoke at 3 am with nausea, and then
vomited and felt dizzy. His dizziness was described
as both lightheadedness and room-spinning.
These symptoms continued for 36 hours before
presentation to the emergency department. He was
diagnosed with viral gastroenteritis, was sent home
with antiemetics, and was advised to maintain
adequate hydration.

On representation to the emergency department,
the patient e notes perseveration of severe
lightheadedness, headache, generalized weakness,
and disequilibrium. The headache is occipital and
pulsatile. The disequilibrium is present primarily
when standing and walking. He feels as though
he will topple over with each step, as though he is
being "pulled to the ground." He denies any other

neurological symptoms. He is known to have had splenic infarcts and portal vein thrombosis in the past. He has no history of hypertension, diabetes, or cigarette smoking.

What do you do now?

CEREBELLAR INFARCT RESULTING FROM BLOOD HYPERVISCOSITY

Discussion Questions

1. Where is the most likely location of his brain lesion?
2. What are the possible underlying causes?
3. What investigations would you undertake?

Discussion

Two weeks after his initial symptoms, the patient returned to his primary care physician, who sent him back to the hospital. Diffusion-weighted brain MRI showed a right cerebellar hemisphere infarct in the territory of the posterior inferior cerebellar artery (Figure 11.1). A magnetic resonance angiogram of the head and neck did not show any vascular stenoses. Cardiac investigation did not reveal any structural or arrhythmia-related causes of brain embolism. Investigations after detection of his splenic infarcts and portal vein thrombosis showed a high red cell count, which was attributed to polycythema vera by a hematologist. During this hospitalization, the patient's hemoglobin level was 16.8 g/dl and hematocrit was 60.6%.

Acute brain infarction and intraparenchymal hemorrhages are potential arterial or venous complications of hyperviscosity syndromes. The clinical presentation of individuals with hyperviscosity syndromes and acute brain infarction does not differ significantly from other etiologies of ischemic stroke. Although many of these infarcts are cortical with apparent neurological deficits, some also may be subcortical with mild or no overt symptoms. The symptoms and deficits of cerebellar infarcts and hemorrhages vary according to lesion location, but most result in loss of coordination (ataxia). Lesions in the lateral aspect of a cerebellar hemisphere cause loss of coordination and muscle tone in the ipsilateral arms and legs (appendicular ataxia), whereas lesions in the vermis and surrounding cerebellar tissue cause loss of postural stability (truncal ataxia) and discoordination of mouth movements. Speech patterns can be altered—slow, irregular, or poorly articulated. Nystagmus (often direction-changing with end gaze) and tremor (especially with movement) are often present.

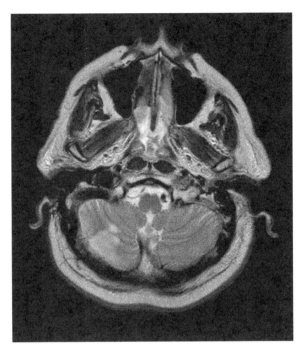

FIGURE 11.1 T2 MRI showing a wedge-shaped, acute right cerebellar infarct in a posterior inferior cerebellar artery territory.

The majority of the following conditions causing hyperviscosity are hemorheologic in nature: sickle cell disease, polycythemia vera, essential thrombocythemia, and more. Concurrent illnesses or circumstances that result in dehydration and volume depletion can lead to thrombosis: vomiting, diarrhea, sweating, excess free water loss through pharmacologic diuresis, and more. In sickle cell disease, ischemic strokes may occur in the setting of pain crises. Thrombosis presumably occurs with in situ thrombosis in the affected end arterioles and venules, although this mechanism is not well established. Sickle cell disease also predisposes individuals to intracranial large-artery stenosis with the development of abnormal collateral vasculature—a nonatherosclerotic vasculopathy also known as *Moyamoya syndrome*. The vast majority of cases of polycythemia vera are related to an activating mutation of Janus kinase 2. Uncommonly, hematologic malignancies including lymphoma, multiple myeloma, and Waldenström's macroglobulinemia can cause ischemic stroke. Although there are several hematologic tests that can detect various forms of hyperviscosity, a complete blood cell count is typically the first commonly obtained laboratory test that detects the relevant abnormalities. Additional blood tests may be needed, such as the genetic screen for Janus kinase 2 in polycythemia vera, fibrinogen, immunophenotyping, and protein electrophoresis of the serum and urine.

The epidemiology of brain infarction and intraparenchymal hemorrhage varies across the age spectrum. For example, brain infarcts are more common in children and older adults with hemoglobin SS, whereas intraparenchymal hemorrhage is more common in young adults in their 20s and 30s. In contrast, polycythemia vera is typically diagnosed in individuals in their 40s to 70s, with mostly thrombotic events (two-thirds arterial and one-third venous). These conditions also confer an inordinately high risk for cerebrovascular conditions. Adults with hemoglobin SS have an incidence of first stroke (ischemic or hemorrhage) of 500 to 1280 per 100,000 person-years compared with 12 to 202 per 100,000 person-years for black adults without sickle cell disease. Nineteen percent of individuals with polycythemia vera in one longitudinal study over 20 years had at least one thrombotic complication; 64% percent preceded the diagnosis of polycythemia vera or occurred at presentation and 36% followed the diagnosis. A similar multicenter study of individuals with polycythemia vera or essential thrombocythemia determined the recurrence risk for thrombosis was 17.7% at 2 years after the first thrombosis, 30.8% at 5 years, and 49.9% at 10 years. The majority of these events were the result of acute brain ischemia—37.4% and 39.7% of initial thrombotic events in polycythemia vera and essential thrombocythemia, respectively, and 42.3% and 35.8% of recurrent thrombotic events, respectively.

The treatment of hyperviscosity syndromes varies by diagnosis but essentially focuses on cytoreduction, hemodilution, and antithrombotic therapy. In sickle cell disease, transfusion therapy (especially exchange transfusion therapy) is an effective treatment, but it is limited by iron overload and alloimmunization. Hydroxyurea is commonly used in both sickle cell disease and myeloproliferative disorders such as polycythemia vera. In polycythemia vera, therapeutic phlebotomies are often scheduled to reduce and maintain the hematocrit level to less than 45%. Both antiplatelet and anticoagulant agents have been used in polycythemia vera, with the former predominantly for arterial thromboses and the latter for venous thromboses.

KEY POINTS TO REMEMBER

- Individuals with hematologic conditions predisposing them to hyperviscosity syndromes are at risk for arterial and venous thrombosis, especially in the setting of illnesses resulting in intravascular volume depletion and hemoconcentration.
- Brain ischemia may be the presentation of polycythemia vera or essential thrombocythemia, or it may precede the diagnosis of these myeloproliferative disorders.
- A complete blood cell count is an important laboratory test in the initial evaluation for acute brain ischemia.
- For polycythemia vera, the optimal treatment strategy for prevention of thrombosis includes therapeutic phlebotomy, hydroxyurea, and antithrombotic medications. It is not yet known whether antiplatelet agents or anticoagulants are preferred; the selection of the antithrombotic agent may depend on an individual's balance of ischemic and hemorrhagic complications.

Further Reading

De Stefano V, Za T, Rossi E, et al. Recurrent thrombosis in patients with polycythemia vera and essential thrombocythemia: incidence, risk factors, and effects of treatments. *Haematologica*. 2008;93:372–380.

Gruppo Italiano Studio Policitemia. Polycythemia vera: the natural history of 1213 patients followed for 20 years. *Ann Intern Med*. 1995;123(9):656–664.

Landolfi R, Marchioli R, Kutti J, et al. Efficacy and safety of low-dose aspirin in polycythemia vera. *N Engl J Med*. 2004;350(2):114–124.

Ohene-Frempong K, Weiner SJ, Sleeper LA, et al. Cerebrovascular accidents in sickle cell disease: rates and risk factors. *Blood*. 1998;91(1):288–294.

Strouse JJ, Lanzkron S, Urrutia V. The epidemiology, evaluation and treatment of stroke in adults with sickle cell disease. *Exp Rev Hematol*. 2011;4(6):597–606.

12 Neck Pain Soon Followed by Right Hemiparesis

Sourabh Lahoti

A 19-year-old right-handed white man presents to the emergency room for sudden development of right-sided weakness, with loss of feeling and slurred speech. The symptoms occurred 30 minutes before arrival while he was working at his desk. He called his roommate, who noted a right facial droop and slurred speech. He was transferred immediately to the emergency room by emergency medical services.

The patient has had pain in his left neck for 1 week. He has never had similar symptoms before. He denies smoking or illicit substance use, and he consumes alcohol in moderation. He does not have hypertension, palpitations, or diabetes.

Examination shows an alert, interactive man with a lean build. His heart rate is regular at 94, his blood pressure is 147/84, and he has a respiratory rate of 20. Auscultation reveals normal heart sounds with no murmurs, good air entry in both lungs, and no bruit over the bilateral carotid and vertebral arteries. Speech is fluent and coherent, but dysarthric. Cranial nerve examination reveals right central facial palsy but is otherwise normal. He has 2/5 strength in the right arm and 4/5 strength in the right leg. Sensation to light touch and pinprick is decreased in the right limbs. Plantar reflex is extensor on the right. He has a National Institutes of Health Stroke Scale score of 6.

What do you do now?

EAGLE'S SYNDROME COMPLICATED BY INTERNAL CAROTID ARTERY DISSECTION AND STROKE

Discussion Questions

1. What is the recommended immediate management?
2. What investigations should be performed?
3. What is the differential diagnosis?
4. What potential alternatives are available to prevent further brain ischemia?

Discussion

Cranial CT was normal. CT angiography showed an irregular 8 × 5-mm outpouching of the left internal carotid artery close to its origin, likely indicative of a pseudoaneurysm (Figure 12.1a). It was adjacent to the tip of the left styloid process, which indented the vessel wall (Figure 12.1b). Complete blood count, metabolic profile, and blood glucose results were all within normal limits. After obtaining informed consent, intravenous tissue plasminogen activator, alteplase, at a dose of 0.9 mg/kg was administered, 10% as a bolus and the rest as an infusion over 1 hour. The infusion was started within 60 minutes of the start of his symptoms and within 20 minutes of his arrival at the hospital.

The patient's symptoms improved by the following day. His speech was normal, and muscle strength was 4/5 in the right arm and 5/5 in the right leg. He was discharged from the hospital 2 days later with complete recovery and no residual deficits.

The left cerebral ischemic episode was attributable to an embolism that arose from the left internal carotid artery dissecting aneurysm. Treatment could involve long-term prophylaxis with antithrombotic agents to prevent thrombus formation within the aneurysmal dilatation. However, this patient is very young, and standard anticoagulants or double antiplatelet treatments pose a substantial risk of bleeding if used over many years. Furthermore, the elongated styloid process could cause recurrent arterial injury. It was decided to gain better views of the arterial lesion, with a potential plan of repairing the aneurysmal lesion and later amputating the styloid process. These alternatives were discussed with the patient and his family.

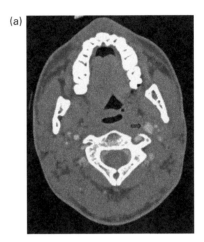

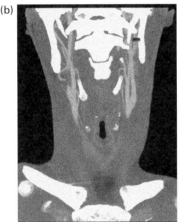

FIGURE 12.1 (a) CT angiogram, axial view, showing an irregular 8 × 5-mm outpouching of the distal left common carotid artery indicative of a pseudoaneurysm (arrow). (b) CT angiogram, coronal view, showing elongated styloid process indenting the left common carotid artery (arrow).

Digital subtraction angiography was done 2 weeks after the stroke. It revealed multiple flaps of dissection in the left internal carotid artery at its origin, with formation of a sizeable pseudoaneurysm. A Viabahn 6 × 25-mm stent graft was placed in the internal carotid artery to exclude the dissection and aneurysm from circulation. Dual antiplatelet therapy with aspirin and clopidogrel was used for long-term stroke prophylaxis. The tip of the styloid process was resected 6 months later by an ear, nose, and throat surgeon.

This case presentation is illustrative of the styloid–carotid artery (Eagle's) syndrome. It is characterized by an abnormally elongated styloid process that compresses the carotid artery, which in turn may lead to dissection, pseudoaneurysm, or both. Dissection leads to formation of thrombi that embolize and may cause distal vessel occlusion and consequent stroke.

This syndrome was first described by Dr. Watt Eagle, an otolaryngeal surgeon, in 1937. It has two forms, one of which is characterized by cervicofacial symptoms of unilateral pharyngeal pain, aggravated by swallowing and frequent reverberation in the ear; it is called *stylohyoid syndrome.* The second clinical syndrome is characterized by compression of the extracranial carotid artery by the elongated styloid process, which leads to arterial dissection and consequent stroke. The elongated styloid process can also impinge on the carotid plexus and may lead to headache and neck pain. In some patients, the styloid process compresses only the carotid artery on lateral flexion of neck to the ipsilateral side. Diagnosis in such individuals is challenging and requires dynamic angiography with and without lateral flexion of the neck. The abnormal styloid process can also compress the jugular vein, leading to thrombosis of the vein and often the lateral sinus that drains into the jugular vein.

Shortening or resection of the styloid process is the recommended treatment. It is a relatively challenging surgery because of the proximity to several important blood vessels, nerves, and muscles to the styloid process.

KEY POINTS TO REMEMBER

· Eagle's syndrome is a rare cause of ischemic stroke through involvement of the carotid artery in the neck by an elongated styloid process.

· Accompanying or preceding nonvascular symptoms include difficulty and pain in swallowing, ear pain, and pain when turning the head toward the ipsilateral side.

· The symptoms are occasionally positional, occurring only on head turning, and the diagnosis in such cases can be challenging, necessitating dynamic angiography.

· Shortening or resecting the elongated styloid process is the recommended treatment.

Further Reading

Farhat HI, Elhammady MS, Ziayee H, Aziz-Sultan MA, Heros RC. Eagle syndrome as a cause of transient ischemic attacks. *J Neurosurg*. 2009;110(1):90–93.

Piagkou M, Anagnostopoulou S, Kouladouros K, Piagkos G. Eagle's syndrome: a review of the literature. *Clin Anat*. 2009;22(5):545–558.

Song J, Ahn S, Cho C. Elongated styloid process as a cause of transient ischemic attacks. *JAMA Neurol*. 2013;70(8):1072–1073.

13 Sudden Onset of Double Vision and Left Ataxic Hemiparesis

Sourabh Lahoti

A 56-year-old right-handed white man had sudden-onset double vision and weakness in his left limbs. He fell while taking a shower and then noted weakness of his left arm and leg. He also developed double vision that was worse on left lateral gaze and resolved after closure of one eye. He could not get up to seek help and was brought to the hospital 20 hours later after his friend found him.

On arrival at the hospital, the patient follows commands, has a regular heart rate of 102, blood pressure of 124/70, and respiration of 20. He is alert and fully oriented, and has fluent, coherent but dysarthric speech. He has a left central facial palsy, left hemiparesis with 4/5 strength in the left arm and leg, and dysmetria of the left arm and leg out of proportion to the hemiparesis. Ocular examination shows anisocoria (mid-size nonreactive right pupil,

normal left pupil), right hypertropia, and exotropia
with limited adduction and depression. Vertical up-
gaze saccades are decreased bilaterally.

His past medical history is significant for
ischemic stroke a year previously, hypertension,
and degenerative spine disease. He has smoked one
pack of cigarettes daily for the past 30 years. He
denies the use of alcohol or illicit drugs.

What do you do now?

MIDBRAIN AND THALAMIC ACUTE INFARCT

Discussion Questions

1. What investigations should be requested?
2. Where is the lesion?
3. What is the most likely cause and the differential diagnosis?

Discussion

Noncontrast head CT showed no acute pathology. There were scattered bihemispheric white matter hypodensities suggestive of chronic ischemic disease. CT angiography revealed occlusion of the right posterior cerebral artery from its proximal segment (Figure 13.1a). Cranial MRI showed an acute right paramedian thalamic and right rostral midbrain infarct (Figure 13.1b). Transthoracic echocardiogram showed normal dimensions of all chambers of the heart, with normal left ventricular ejection fraction and no intracardiac thrombus.

This case illustrates a rostral mesencephalic–medial thalamic stroke syndrome. The rostral midbrain and medial thalamus have a common blood supply from the paramedian mesencephalic perforating arteries that originate from the proximal segment of the posterior cerebral artery. This patient has the clinical syndromes contralateral ataxic hemiparesis, ipsilateral incomplete third nerve palsy, and bilateral up-gaze palsy.

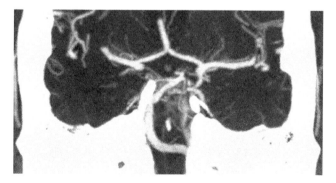

FIGURE 13.1   CT angiogram, coronal view, showing abrupt termination of right posterior cerebral artery shortly after its origin from the basilar artery). The left posterior cerebral artery arises from the posterior communicating artery. The basilar artery is tortuous and has luminal irregularity, which is suggestive of atherosclerotic disease.

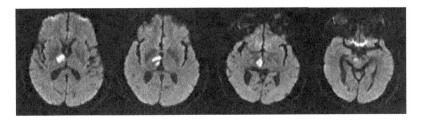

FIGURE 13.2 Diffusion-weighted brain MRI showing restricted diffusion in the right medial thalamus and the right side of the rostral midbrain.

The ataxic hemiparesis was caused by disruption of the corticospinal and corticopontine fibers in the cerebral peduncle. Third nerve palsy was caused by disruption of the third nerve fibers as they traversed through the midbrain. There was ipsilateral adduction, supraduction, and infraduction palsy, with dilatation of pupil and loss of pupillary response, but without ptosis. The mesencephalic course of the third nerve is organized into three groups of fascicles: rostral, intermediate, and caudal. The rostral group contains fibers to the sphincter pupillae and inferior rectus, the intermediate group has fibers to the medial rectus and inferior oblique, and the caudal group contains fibers to the superior rectus and levator palpebrae superioris. Sparing of the levator palpebrae superioris is probably because of the most caudal location or different blood supply of the caudal fascicle by lateral branches of the same perforating arteries, whereas the rostral and intermediate fascicles are supplied from medial branches. Bilateral up-gaze palsy is probably secondary to the disruption of the frontocortical fibers responsible for supranuclear control of the ventral gaze as they traverse through the medial thalamus, or the result of the lesion of the rostral interstitial nucleus of the medial longitudinal fasciculus, which is involved in generating vertical saccades. Saccadic innervation is unilateral to the depressor muscles but bilateral to the elevator muscles.

Similar but slightly different syndromes known widely in the neuroanatomy and clinical neurology literature, with their eponymous names, arise from strokes in the area of the ventral midbrain supplied by the perforating arteries stemming from the tip of the basilar artery and the proximal posterior cerebral artery. It should be emphasized they constitute variations on the same theme and reflect different degrees of involvement of neighboring anatomic structures. In addition to the (*ipsilateral*) third nerve, which is a common denominator, contralateral hemiparesis and contralateral hemiataxia can be seen.

Contralateral hemiparesis is a result of the involvement of the cortico-pontine and corticospinal fibers in the cerebral peduncle running in the ventral surface of the midbrain. When hemiparesis dominates the clinical picture, the clinical syndrome is often referred to as *Weber's syndrome.*

Contralateral hemiataxia is another commonly seen feature that results from the involvement of the adjacently located superior cerebellar peduncle. A distinct coarse, slow tremor (known as *rubral tremor*) ensues as a result of the involvement of the red nucleus. Claude's and Benedikt's syndrome have been used in the nomenclature and, although they are described as distinct entities, they cause more confusion than diagnostic clarity. In reality, the clinical picture is usually a mix, in varying degrees, of all the previously mentioned symptoms and signs. Strokes in the area of the rostral midbrain area can be a result of small penetrating vessel disease or a thrombus at the tip of the basilar artery. The latter might herald potentially life-threatening conditions such as basilar artery thrombosis and should be managed accordingly.

KEY POINTS TO REMEMBER

· Strokes in the area of the rostral midbrain and thalamus can cause a number of similar, but slightly different, clinical syndromes, with the main features of ipsilateral third nerve palsy, and contralateral hemiparesis and hemiataxia in differing degrees.

· Additional signs such as supranuclear vertical gaze palsies can be seen, depending on the exact anatomic structures involved.

· The vessels involved are small perforating vessels that stem from the proximal part of the posterior cerebral artery or the very distal part of the basilar artery.

· Some of the syndromes are known with eponymous names; these terms should be used more as crude guides to the clinical syndrome because they are rarely seen in their pure "textbook" form.

Further Reading

Ahdab R, Riachi N. Vertical "half-and-a-half" syndrome. *J Neurol Neurosurg Psychiatry*. 2012;83:834–835.

Bhidayasiri R, Plant GT, Leigh RJ. A hypothetical scheme for the brainstem control of vertical gaze. *Neurology*. 2000;54(10):1985–1993.

Bogousslavsky J, Regli F. Upgaze palsy and monocular paresis of downward gaze from ipsilateral thalamo-mesencephalic infarction: a vertical "one-and-a-half" syndrome. *J Neurol*. 1984;231:43–45.

Buttner-Ennever J, Buttner U, Cohen B, Baumgartner G. Vertical gaze paralysis and the rostral interstitial nucleus of the medial longitudinal fasciculus. *Brain*. 1982;105:125–149.

Clark JM, Albers GW. Vertical gaze palsies from medial thalamic infarctions without midbrain involvement. *Stroke*. 1995;26(8):1467–1470.

Vitošević Z, Marinković S, Cetković M, et al. Intramesencephalic course of the oculomotor nerve fibers: microanatomy and possible clinical significance. *Anat Sci Int*. 2013;88(2):70–82.

14 Arm Pain and Swelling Followed by Headache, Right Weakness, and Aphasia

Louis R. Caplan

A 51-year-old left-handed woman presented with worsening headache and right-limb dysfunction. After she developed persistent arm pain and swelling, she was found to have a left-arm blood clot. She initially applied hot compresses, but after seeing multiple doctors she was started on warfarin 5 days later.

On August 1st, she bumped her head and began to report right-sided headaches. Cranial CT was negative for blood. The headaches became more severe and persistent, and she developed nausea, became sleepier, and reported that her right thumb was numb. As her friends prepared to bring her to the hospital they noted her right limbs were weak. She was admitted to the hospital on August 18.

Her past history includes a myocardial infarct at the age of 40. Examination shows a somnolent woman with nonfluent perseverative speech. Her right face is flattened, she cannot move her right arm, and her right leg is quite weak. She localizes stimuli well on her right limbs, and her right plantar response is extensor. A CT scan taken on the day of admission shows a hemorrhagic lesion involving the left cerebral hemisphere.

What do you do now?

CEREBRAL VENOUS SINUS THROMBOSIS PRESENTING WITH HEMORRHAGE AND BRAIN EDEMA

Discussion Questions

1. What is the most likely diagnosis?
2. What are other likely differential diagnoses?

Discussion

As mentioned, a CT scan taken on the day of admission showed a hemorrhagic lesion involving the left cerebral hemisphere (Figure 14.1a).

The often-cited advice concerning patients on anticoagulants is that it is essential to stop the anticoagulant and even reverse its function when important bleeding develops. The key differential diagnostic concerns in this patient are (1) intracerebral hemorrhage attributed to warfarin and (2) cerebral venous thrombosis (CVT).

The physicians caring for her followed the "knee-jerk" response and stopped the warfarin, then gave her osmotic therapy to decrease brain edema. Three days later, she became comatose and her left plantar response became extensor. MRI now showed more extensive abnormalities in the posterior left cerebral hemisphere (Figure 14.1b). and a new right cerebral hypodensity. Magnetic resonance venograam showed a left lateral sinus and superior sagittal sinus occlusions. She was treated with heparin followed by warfarin. A hemicraniectomy was performed. Additional

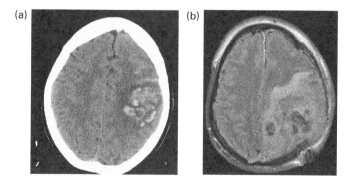

FIGURE 14.1 (a) Noncontrast head CT with left frontal convexity hemorrhage with adjacent parenchymal hypodensity. (b) Brain MRI with cerebral edema (hyperintense part) and hemorrhagic component (hypointense part).

evaluation showed the patient had a lupus anticoagulant and positive anti-cardiolipin antibodies.

The clues to the correct diagnosis in this case were there from the beginning: (1) arm venous thrombosis, (2) prior myocardial infarct at age 40, and (3) CT scan (Figure 14.1a) showing edema and scattered hemorrhages unlike the usual, homogeneous, well-circumscribed hematoma related to warfarin bleeding. Had these clues been recognized, CT venography or magnetic resonance venography could have been performed to clarify the diagnosis, and anticoagulants could have been continued (acceptable treatment for CVT with intracranial bleeding).

During the ensuing weeks, the patient's clinical signs improved and she, ultimately, was able to return to work. Because much of the parenchymal abnormalities in patients with cerebral venous thrombosis are attributable to reversible brain edema, the prognosis in these patients is often good.

KEY POINTS TO REMEMBER

· Not every intracerebral hemorrhage mandates anticoagulation cessation or reversal.
· CVT often presents with hemorrhagic changes.
· Despite the presence of hemorrhagic changes, anticoagulation remains the mainstay of treatment for CVT.
· It is important that CVT be kept in the differential diagnosis because its management is diametrically different than that of other causes of intracerebral hemorrhage, and delay in treatment can be fatal.

Further Reading

Antiphospholipid Antibodies in Stroke Study (APASS) Group. Clinical and laboratory findings in patients with antiphospholipid antibodies and cerebral ischemia. *Stroke.* 1990;21:1268–1273.

Caplan LR, Bousser M-G. Cerebral venous thrombosis. In Caplan LR, ed. *Caplan's Stroke.* 5th ed. Cambridge: Cambridge University Press; 2016.

Cervera R, Piette JC, Font J, et al. Antiphospholipid syndrome: clinical and immunologic manifestations and patterns of disease expression in a cohort of 1,000 patients. *Arthritis Rheum.* 2002;46:1019–1027.

Feldmann E, Levine SR. Cerebrovascular disease with antiphospholipid
    antibodies: immune mechanisms, significance, and therapeutic options. *Ann
    Neurol.* 1995;37(suppl 1):S114–S130.
Roldan J, Brey RL. Antiphospholipid antibody syndrome. In Caplan LR, ed.
    Uncommon Causes of Stroke. 2nd ed. Cambridge: Cambridge University
    Press; 2008:263–274.
Verro P, Levine SR, Tietjen GE. Cerebrovascular ischemic events with high positive
    anticardiolipin antibodies. *Stroke.* 1998;29:2245–2253.

15 More Than Meets the Eye

Vasileios-Arsenios Lioutas

A 41-year-old right-handed white woman presents
to the neurology clinic for evaluation of a visual
disturbance. She has a known, long-standing
history of migraine with aura; her headaches
are stereotyped, preceded by visual aura
with scintillating scotomata, accompanied by
photosensitivity and nausea, which resolve with
triptan use and rest. Four days before the clinic
visit, the patient experienced what seemed to be the
beginning of a typical migraine attack; however, the
headache did not respond as promptly to triptan.
Although her aura subsided and the patient had no
difficulty seeing, and she could identify individual
letters, reading words or sentences was initially
almost impossible and subsequently unusually
laborious for her. The headache eventually
subsided, but she reports a lingering difficulty
reading. She takes no medications besides the
occasional triptan. On examination, she has intact
visual fields, strength, sensorium, and coordination.

She can write without difficulty. In general, she reads fluently, but with some hesitancy, and experiences obvious difficulty for longer or unfamiliar words.

What do you do now?

ALEXIA WITHOUT AGRAPHIA IN A YOUNG WOMAN WITH COMPLEX MIGRAINES

Discussion Questions

1. Is there reason to be concerned for something more serious than a migraine aura?
2. Is there any link between migraine and stroke?
3. What is the neuroanatomic localization of the patient's symptoms and clinical examination findings?
4. Is there a need for additional workup?

Discussion

This is a young woman with frequent complex migraines with stereotyped visual auras. Several features in her presentation are alarming. The duration of her current visual symptoms is unusually long. Migraine aura typically precedes the headache, although on occasion it might occur concurrently or even after it; but, by definition, its duration does not exceed 60 minutes—or a maximum of a few hours in extreme cases. This patient's symptoms have persisted for more than 4 days and have outlived the headache, which is a rather unusual feature for a migrainous aura. In addition, the nature of the visual symptoms is concerning. Migrainous visual auras as usually described as positive visual phenomena with zigzag lines, bright straight lines, circles, or other elemental shapes as a result of activation of the occipital cortex. This activation is followed by a slowly spreading wave of neuronal suppression, known as *cortical spreading depression*, which is believed to the pathophysiologic basis of the migrainous aura.

This patient's deficits are dramatically different. She is able to write fluently and can recognize individual letters, but she has difficulty recognizing letter sequences as words and sentences. This clinical syndrome is known as *pure alexia* or, alternatively, *alexia without agraphia*. Neuroanatomically, it occurs from involvement of the dominant occipital cortex and parasplenial area, with vascular supply from the posterior cerebral artery. It results in a disconnection syndrome between the visual cortex and the language centers, which explains the difficulty recognizing written language. Brain MRI was conducted urgently in this patient and revealed a left parieto-occipital infarct, compatible with her clinical deficit (Figure 15.1).

The relationship between migraine and stroke is complex. Epidemiologic studies confirm a relative risk for ischemic stroke of approximately 2.2, with the relationship being more robust in migraine with aura. Smoking and oral contraceptive use add significant excessive risk, nearly tripling it to 7 to 8. The underlying pathophysiologic link is not well understood and it should be noted that, despite doubling the risk, in absolute terms stroke remains a rare event in people with migraine, and therefore there is no justification for additional workup or precautions in migraineurs, beyond control of concurrent cardiovascular risk factors if present.

On clinical grounds, differentiation between a migraine aura and a transient ischemic attack can be challenging. Migraine aura can take many different forms beyond the classic scintillating scotoma, presenting as a sensory disturbance, motor weakness, and language difficulties, among others. The rate of symptom progression is a key distinguishing feature. Migrainous aura symptoms build up gradually, following a "marching"

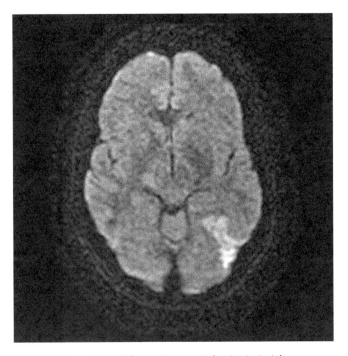

FIGURE 15.1   Diffusion-weighted MRI revealing acute infarction in the left temporo-occipital area.

pattern over several minutes, perhaps mirroring the spreading wave of cortical depression. In contrast, symptoms resulting from a vascular event present abruptly, within seconds. The mode of symptom resolution is similar. Therefore, an abrupt rate of onset, atypical for the patient's symptoms, and an unusually prolonged duration of symptoms are grounds for concern and further workup.

Migraine patients with ischemic stroke should receive a thorough workup, similar to any other stroke patient, to identify underlying treatable causes. "Migrainous infarction," referring to an ischemic stroke in the context of an unusually prolonged migraine attack, is a rare entity and should be a diagnosis of exclusion. In this young adult with ischemic stroke, the patient should receive thorough vessel imaging of the neck and head, including the aortic arch, and a laboratory workup, including a hypercoagulability panel. A thorough review of medications, including oral contraceptive medications, and personal and family history is key. A transthoracic echocardiogram with a low threshold to proceed with a transesophageal study to detect possible structural heart defects, such as a patent foramen ovale, are very important. Any additional workups should be tailored to the findings (or lack thereof) of the initial workup. Low-dose aspirin daily is a reasonable, initial secondary prevention choice, pending completion of the stroke workup.

KEY POINTS TO REMEMBER

- Migraine is associated with a poorly understood and approximately twofold relative risk of ischemic stroke; but, in absolute terms, stroke in migraineurs is rare.
- Migraine aura can be difficult to distinguish from a transient ischemic attack at times, but details such the rate of onset and symptom duration might offer useful clues.
- Migraine patients with ischemic stroke should receive a full and thorough workup, similar to any other stroke patient

---

Further Reading

Bousser MG, Welch KM. Relation between migraine and stroke. *Lancet Neurol.* 2005;4(9):533–542.

Ferro JM, Massaro AR, Mas JL. Aetiological diagnosis of ischaemic stroke in young adults. *Lancet Neurol.* 2010;9(11):1085–1096.

Kurth T, Chabriat H, Bousser MG. Migraine and stroke: a complex association with clinical implications. *Lancet Neurol.* 2012;11(1):92–100.

Leff AP, Behrmann M. Treatment of reading impairment after stroke. *Curr Opin Neurol.* 2008;21(6):644–648.

Starrfelt R, Olafsdóttir RR, Arendt IM. Rehabilitation of pure alexia: a review. *Neuropsychol Rehabil.* 2013;23(5):755–779.

16   A Rusty Pipe

Vasileios-Arsenios Lioutas

A 66-year-old right-handed black man presents
to the emergency room with sudden onset of
difficulty speaking and right hand weakness.
He has a history of inadequately controlled
hypertension and hypercholesterolemia,
and a 35 pack-year history of smoking. His
medications include 20 mg atorvastatin and
81 mg aspirin started 3 weeks earlier for a
transient ischemic attack (TIA) with symptoms
identical to his current presentation.

   On examination, his blood pressure is 151/85, and
he is afebrile and fully alert. His speech is halted,
with frequent pauses to find the appropriate word,
and he has difficulty naming low-frequency objects.
His repetition and ability to follow commands are
intact. Visual fields, sensorium, and strength are
intact, with the exception of clumsiness and mild
weakness of the right hand. A noncontrast head
CT is unremarkable, and a rapid evaluation of his
extracranial internal carotid arteries with ultrasound

reveals minimal (<30%) stenosis. A transthoracic echocardiogram and continuous heart monitor from his recent hospitalization do not reveal any relevant culprits.

RECURRENT ISCHEMIC STROKES RESULTING FROM INTRACRANIAL ATHEROSCLEROTIC DISEASE

Discussion Questions

1. What is the possible anatomic localization of this patient's symptoms?
2. What additional workup is necessary?
3. What is the optimal management approach?

Discussion

This patient has symptoms that localize to the left middle cerebral artery (MCA) territory. His language deficit pattern is characterized by expressive and naming difficulties with preserved comprehension and repetition. This deficit pattern is known as *transcortical motor aphasia* and it localizes to the dominant anterior frontal lobe, usually in a subcortical area adjacent to, but sparing, the Broca's area in the anterior inferior frontal cortex. The pattern of his weakness involving the hand primarily suggests a discrete, focal lesion in the contralateral motor cortex or, alternatively, part of the descending motor fibers before they converge to form the internal capsule. Taken together, this patient's clinical findings suggest at least two distinct lesions within the left MCA territory. Indeed, his brain MRI reveals acute infarctions within the left frontal lobe (Figure 16.1a).

The next issue that needs to be addressed is the possible underlying etiology of these strokes. Cardioembolism from paroxysmal atrial fibrillation or a cardiac thrombus is a consideration. However, the patient's transthoracic echocardiogram excluded a structural cardiac lesion and his long-term heart monitor makes atrial fibrillation less likely, although it does not exclude it entirely. There is a detail in the patient's history that merits special attention: he had a TIA with similar symptoms, referable to the same vascular territory, which should focus attention to the possibility of a fixed vascular lesion as the source. One additional detail favoring a site of arterial thrombosis as an embolic source is the appearance of the acute infarcts on the MRI. Arterial atherosclerotic plaques are more likely to result in small, distal infarcts, in contrast to cardioembolic infarcts, which tend to occlude major vessels and result in larger territorial infarctions.

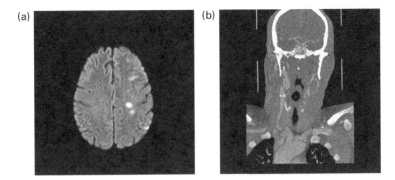

FIGURE 16.1 (a) Diffusion-weighted MRI shows acute infarctions in the left frontal lobe in a territory supplied by the middle cerebral artery (MCA). (b) Coronal sections of the CT angiogram. Notice the high-grade stenosis in the proximal segment of the left MCA.

The patient's carotid ultrasound excludes the possibility of an extra-cranial internal carotid artery stenosis, so the logical next step is to search for a lesion in the left MCA. A vascular study, either magnetic resonance angiography or CT angiography should be obtained. CT angiography in this case confirmed the presence of stenosis and an irregularity in the proximal segment of the left MCA (Figure 16.1b) suggestive of in situ atherosclerosis, which likely accounts for the recurrent TIA and ischemic stroke.

Intracranial atherosclerotic disease (ICAD) accounts for approximately 10% of the ischemic strokes and TIAs in the United States. Its population-wide prevalence is not well known, but it affects blacks and Asians more than whites, for reasons that are not well understood. Mechanisms by which ICAD can cause a stroke include distal artery-to-artery embolism, in situ complete thrombotic occlusion, hemodynamic compromise and hypoperfusion in severe stenosis, and, last, obstruction of the orifice of penetrating vessels originating from the parent vessel at the site of athero-sclerotic plaque formation. Of these mechanisms, distal arterial embolism is by far the most common. Hypoperfusion-related ischemia, leading to border-zone or "watershed" infarcts, occurs but it is less common than generally perceived. Significant and prolonged hypotension, in conjunc-tion with a poor collateral network, are necessary to cause a stroke through this mechanism.

The management of symptomatic ICAD has been studied in several trials during the past decade. Artery angioplasty and stenting does not constitute standard of care and is generally not offered, with rare exceptions of cases refractory to medical management. The accepted optimal medical management includes a combination of aspirin and clopidogrel along with high-dose statin and aggressive optimization of other risk factors, such as diabetes, hypertension, smoking, and lack of exercise. The efficacy of dual antiplatelet treatment beyond 3 months is not well established; in general, long-term dual antiplatelet therapy is not recommended for secondary stroke prevention. Anticoagulation with warfarin was not found superior to aspirin in a large trial and, as such, it does not constitute standard of care, although it might be used as an alternative option in cases of antiplatelet failure.

KEY POINTS TO REMEMBER

- ICAD accounts for approximately 10% of ischemic strokes in the United States, and affects Asians and blacks disproportionately.
- The most common mechanism by which ICAD causes stroke is through artery-to-artery embolism.
- Angioplasty and stenting have no proven efficacy and are not offered routinely.
- A combination of aspirin and clopidogrel accompanied by a high-dose statin is a reasonable regimen for secondary prevention of strokes secondary to symptomatic ICAD.
- Aggressive control of cardiovascular risk factors, healthy diet, and exercise are also key features of lowering recurrent stroke risk.

Further Reading

Chimowitz MI, Lynn MJ, Derdeyn CP, et al. Stenting versus aggressive medical therapy for intracranial arterial stenosis. *N Engl J Med.* 2011;365(11):993–1003.

Chimowitz MI, Lynn MJ, Howlett-Smith H, et al. Comparison of warfarin and aspirin for symptomatic intracranial arterial stenosis. *N Engl J Med.* 2005;352(13):1305–1316.

Derdeyn CP, Chimowitz MI, Lynn MJ, et al. Aggressive medical treatment
     with or without stenting in high-risk patients with intracranial artery
     stenosis (SAMMPRIS): the final results of a randomised trial. *Lancet*.
     2014;383(9914):333–341.

Gonzalez NR, Liebeskind DS, Dusick JR, Mayor F, Saver J. Intracranial arterial
     stenoses: current viewpoints, novel approaches, and surgical perspectives.
     Neurosurg Rev. 2013;36(2):175–184.

Holmstedt CA, Turan TN, Chimowitz MI. Atherosclerotic intracranial
     arterial stenosis: risk factors, diagnosis, and treatment. *Lancet Neurol*.
     2013;12(11):1106–1114.

López-Cancio E, Matheus MG, Romano JG, et al. Infarct patterns, collaterals
     and likely causative mechanisms of stroke in symptomatic intracranial
     atherosclerosis. *Cerebrovasc Dis*. 2014;37(6):417–422.

17 Eyelid Droopiness and Body Weakness

Luciana Catanese

A 52-year-old right-handed man without any significant past medical history presents for evaluation of intense headache and neck pain that has lasted for several days. The patient had noticed right eye droopiness, and his left arm and leg felt heavy, which led him to the emergency room. He complains of a dull pain in the right side of his neck, which he had attributed to a pulled muscle and tried to treat with hot compresses and over-the-counter analgesics to no effect. The headache occurred rather abruptly and is described as very intense and throbbing. Examination reveals normal blood pressure and temperature, with a sinus tachycardia. The patient is in acute distress, secondary to significant right-sided neck pain, with accompanying right-sided ptosis, miosis, subtle left facial weakness with sparing of the forehead, and pronator drift of the left arm. He denies any recent history of trauma, neck manipulation, or other neurological symptoms. He indicates that he lifts heavy boxes on a daily basis as part of his job. He takes no medications nor does he smoke or use alcohol or illicit drugs.

What do you do now?

RIGHT INTERNAL CAROTID ARTERY DISSECTION

Discussion Questions

1. Based on this patient's presentation, where would you localize the lesion?
2. What is the most likely mechanism of stroke?
3. What imaging studies would you order based on the patient's symptoms?
4. What is a common radiographic finding in this condition?
5. For how long would you treat this patient?

Discussion

The main features of this case are thunderclap headache followed by right Horner's syndrome, and left-sided facial and brachial paresis. Facial weakness with sparing of the forehead is seen with lesions involving the contralateral corticobulbar tract above the level of the cranial nerve VII nucleus in the pons. The forehead is spared in unilateral lesions above this level as a result of bilateral cortical representation. Pronator drift is a sensitive test for subtle weakness resulting from lesions of the contralateral corticospinal tract. Considering the absence of cortical signs such as neglect, agnosia, apraxia, aphasia, or visual field defects, the causative lesion is likely a subcortical one that involves the corticobulbar and spinal tracts. The patient's MRI demonstrates multiple cortical and subcortical embolic-appearing infarcts within the territory of the right middle cerebral artery (Figure 17.1a). Because of the contiguous representation of the arm and face in the motor cortices and pathways, the concomitant involvement of face and arm is a common clinical finding. All the symptoms mentioned previously are related to brain ischemia, but some symptoms can be related purely to an arterial wall lesion. They include neck pain and Horner's syndrome, as seen in this patient, although pulsatile tinnitus and loss of function of the lower cranial nerves (IX–XII) can also be seen. The combination of ptosis, miosis, and hemianhidrosis is known as *Horner's syndrome*. This syndrome results from a lesion along the sympathetic fibers supplying the superior tarsal muscle in the eyelid, the pupillary dilator muscle, and sweat glands in the face, and it can result from strategic lesions anywhere from the brainstem to the orbit. However, the lack of anhidrosis in this case localizes the lesion to the carotid sympathetic plexus above the carotid bifurcation where the sudomotor fibers to the face take off.

Horner's syndrome with accompanying headache and neck pain should, however, raise concerns for underlying carotid arterial dissection. Dissections are tears in the middle coat of the arteries that can be either traumatic or spontaneous. Some conditions, such as acquired or congenital connective tissue disorders, can make individuals more vulnerable to dissections, but most patients with dissection do not have concurrent

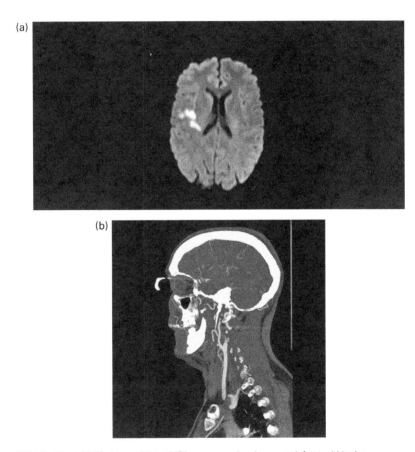

FIGURE 17.1 (a) Diffusion-weighted MRI sequence showing acute infarct within the right middle cerebral artery territory. (b) Sagittal view of CT angiogram of the neck with a characteristic "flame-shaped" tapering of the right proximal internal carotid artery, which is strongly suggestive of dissection.

disorders, as seen in this patient. In the case of the carotid artery, this is the second most common lesion after atherosclerosis. Traumatic dissections can result from what may seem trivial activity, such as heavy lifting. This patient experienced a right internal carotid artery dissection leading to complete occlusion of the carotid artery (Figure 17.1b) and subsequent thromboembolism into the middle cerebral artery. The posited explanation for the occurrence of distal embolization in this condition is that the spreading of arterial wall disruption into the intimal surface of the vessel allows for partially coagulated blood to enter the lumen and travel distally. Acute narrowing of the lumen by an expansive intramural clot can also lead to brain ischemia resulting from cerebral hypoperfusion, emboli, or both.

CT angiography and magnetic resonance angiography are the preferred diagnostic modalities because of their noninvasive nature and fast acquisition times. The characteristic radiographic finding is the "flame sign," which represents a tapering occlusion. Antiplatelet therapy for 3 to 6 months is the preferred treatment for this condition. However, anticoagulation is an appropriate treatment alternative for preventing strokes in the acute setting, considering the lack of evidence to support an increase in the risk of bleeding or increased extent of the dissection—a major longstanding theoretical concern in this population. In the absence of clinical trial data for guidance, the duration of treatment is dictated by the estimated time of healing of the arterial wall.

KEY POINTS TO REMEMBER

- The coexistence of Horner's syndrome, headache, and neck pain should raise suspicion for arterial dissection.
- The mechanism of stroke in arterial dissection is most commonly related to distal embolization from the site of arterial wall disruption.
- The "flame sign" is a common radiographic finding in this condition.
- Antiplatelet therapy for 3 to 6 months is the preferred treatment modality. Anticoagulation can be considered in the acute setting.

Further Reading

Blumenfeld H. *Neuroanatomy through Clinical Cases*. 2nd ed.

Caplan CR. *Vertebrobasilar Ischemia and Hemorrhage: Clinical Findings, Diagnosis and Management of Posterior Circulation Disease*. 2nd ed.

Caplan CR. *Caplan's Stroke: A Clinical Approach*. 4th ed.

Markus HS. Antiplatelet treatment compared with anticoagulation treatment for cervical artery dissection (CADISS): a randomized trial. *Lancet Neurol*. 2015;14:361–367.

18 A Pain in the Hand

Vasileios-Arsenios Lioutas

A 67-year-old right-handed woman presents
to the emergency room with acute onset of
pain in her left hand and leg. She was in her
usual state of health until the acute onset of
an intense but difficult-to-describe painful
sensation in her left hemibody, which is
particularly intense in her hand. She noticed no
other symptoms. She has a history of poorly
controlled hypertension, but no other medical
issues. Her medications include lisinopril and
simvastatin.

On examination, the patient has a blood pressure
of 168/98. She is lying on the stretcher in moderate
discomfort and she is anxious. She is fully oriented,
with intact language. Her coordination is intact and
she has her strength full, with the exception of the
left hand, which is kept in a strange posture: flexed
in the wrist and metacarpophalangeal joints. On
sensory examination, she has a disproportionate
reaction to simple touch on her left side, especially

in the hand and forearm area, which she describes as extremely sensitive. An urgent noncontrast head CT does not reveal acute hemorrhage, ischemia, or other intracranial process.

What do you do now?

RIGHT LATERAL THALAMIC STROKE WITH ALLODYNIA/ PAIN AS THE ACUTE PRESENTING SYMPTOM

Discussion Questions

1. What does the patient's clinical presentation suggest?
2. What additional workup, if any, is necessary?
3. What is the prognosis of her condition?
4. What is the indicated treatment?

Discussion

This patient's presentation is puzzling at first and, indeed, her discomfort and anxiety initially raise concern for anxiety attack or somatization. However, a closer inspection of her symptoms and examination findings tells a different story. Her sensory deficit is described as allodynia, which is a term used to describe an altered sensory perception, which evokes a noxious sensation in response to a naturally nonnoxious stimulus, such as light touch or temperature. This usually occurs as a result of central pain sensitization, often in response to repetitive painful stimulation, such as in the case of complex regional pain syndrome or cutaneous allodynia that affects the skin of the scalp or face in patients with chronic migraine. In this case, however, there is no history of repetitive painful stimulation and, most important, the symptoms started abruptly. The mode of presentation suggests either an acute mechanical injury or a vascular event, migraine, or epileptic phenomenon. The latter two are not likely, given no prior history of migraine or epilepsy and mode of presentation; symptoms usually culminate over several seconds or minutes, following a marching pattern. There is no recent or remote history of neck injury, and the anatomic distribution of symptoms does not fit a radicular or peripheral nerve pattern. There is an additional aspect of the patient's examination that is particularly useful if taken into account. The left hand posture, although neglected initially as simply strange, can in fact be seen as a result of thalamic infarctions and is known as *thalamic hand*, which is, in essence, a dystonic posture of the hand resulting from disruption in the thalamic–basal ganglia–motor cortex feedback loop.

Additional workup is necessary, and the patient received a brain MRI, which revealed a small infarct in the right lateral thalamus (Figure 18.1). These infarctions are often classified as "lacunar" infarcts and result from small penetrating vessel disease. The underlying process is usually a slowly progressive structural change in the vessel wall, known as *lipohyalinosis*, resulting from the cumulative effect of chronic exposure to cardiovascular risk factors such as hypertension and diabetes. The affected vessel in this particular case appears to be the thalamogeniculate artery, a small vessel originating from the posterior cerebral artery. An embolic occlusion from a more proximal source such as the heart, or an atherosclerotic plaque in the vertebral artery or the aortic arch are also considerations, and this patient should receive a full workup, including vessel and cardiac imaging and laboratory studies.

This patient's presentation is an atypical presentation of thalamic pain syndrome, also known as *Dejerine-Roussy syndrome*, from the names of the two French neurologists who first described it in 1906. The syndrome results from an infarct in the lateral thalamus disrupting the spinothalamic tract that conveys sensory stimuli to the somatosensory cortex. This patient's presentation is atypical in the sense that the pain and allodynia almost always develop as a delayed, chronic effect, usually several months after the infarct. The initial sensory symptoms usually involve numbness or paresthesias in the contralateral face, arm, and leg.

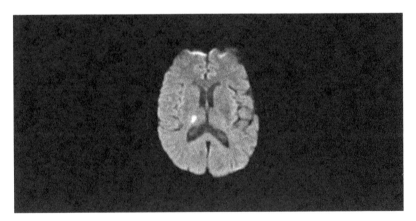

FIGURE 18.1 Diffusion-weighted MRI showing acute infarct in the right posterolateral thalamus.

Although linked traditionally with thalamic strokes, central pain syndrome is not exclusive to the thalamus or to strokes only. Any lesion along the spinothalamic tract, disrupting the transmission of sensory information from the periphery to the somatosensory cortex, can result in such a problem. Its management poses a significant challenge. Several agents and approaches have been used, including gabapentin, pregabalin, opiates, non-steroidal anti-inflammatory analgesics, anticonvulsants, local lidocaine, and sympathetic blocks, but the symptoms are generally refractory and difficult to control. Nonpharmacologic interventions such as biofeedback technique and acupuncture might be considered in particularly refractory cases. In the case of ischemic stroke, addressing comorbid conditions, such as depression, concurrent arthritic pain and spasticity can offer significant relief.

KEY POINTS TO REMEMBER

- Lateral thalamic infarcts can result in chronic allodynia and neuropathic pain in the contralateral face, arm, or leg.
- In the vast majority of cases, pain occurs as a late manifestation, several months after the initial insult.
- Poststroke pain is difficult to manage; control of comorbidities such as depression, spasticity, and arthritic pain is important in reducing patient discomfort.

Further Reading

Frese A, Husstedt IW, Ringelstein EB, Evers S. Pharmacologic treatment of central post-stroke pain. *Clin J Pain.* 2006;22(3):252–260.

Georgiadis AL, Yamamoto Y, Kwan ES, Pessin MS, Caplan LR. Anatomy of sensory findings in patients with posterior cerebral artery territory infarction. *Arch Neurol.* 1999;56(7):835–838.

Harrison RA, Field TS. Post stroke pain: identification, assessment, and therapy. *Cerebrovasc Dis.* 2015;39(3–4):190–201.

Klit H, Finnerup NB, Jensen TS. Central post-stroke pain: clinical characteristics, pathophysiology, and management. *Lancet Neurol.* 2009;8(9):857–868.

Nicholson BD. Evaluation and treatment of central pain syndromes. *Neurology.* 2004;62(5)(suppl 2):S30–S36.

Schmahmann JD. Vascular syndromes of the thalamus. *Stroke.* 2003;34(9):2264–2278.

19 A Ticking Time Bomb

Vasileios-Arsenios Lioutas

A 72-year-old right-handed man presents for
evaluation of left face and arm weakness that
started abruptly several hours earlier. He quit
smoking 2 years previously, after a 40-pack
year history, and has a history of peripheral
vascular disease, hypercholesterolemia, and
hypertension. His medications include low-
dose aspirin, 80 mg atorvastatin, and lisinopril.
He adds that he has had two episodes with
similar symptoms of left face and arm
weakness during the past week that resolved
spontaneously, and an additional episode of
what he describes as "vision in the right eye
going black" for several minutes 4 days earlier.
On examination, his blood pressure is 135/
96. He is alert, converses without difficulty,
and has intact visual fields and sensation.
His speech is dysarthric and his left face and
arm are weak, with marked clumsiness of the
left hand, although his left leg is spared. He

denies headache or recent trauma. There is
no bruit on carotid auscultation. He claims full
compliance with all his medications.

What do you do now?

SYMPTOMATIC RIGHT INTERNAL CAROTID ARTERY STENOSIS

Discussion Questions

1. What is the possible anatomic localization of the patient's symptoms and for which underlying pathophysiologic process do they raise concern?
2. What additional workup is necessary?
3. How should this patient be treated?

Discussion

This patient reports motor symptoms affecting primarily his face and arm, sparing the leg. This suggests involvement of areas involving and adjacent to the right primary motor cortex. His symptoms also suggest involvement of middle cerebral artery branches only, because the lower limb motor cortex area is supplied by the anterior cerebral artery. A small subcortical infarct sparing a part of the white matter tract responsible for leg movements is theoretically plausible, but unlikely. Careful examination might reveal subtle signs that are often overlooked, such as agraphesthesia extinction of simultaneous sensory stimuli, the presence of which can offer additional cues to a possible cortical as opposed to subcortical location. Obviously, in a large hemispheric stroke, all these symptoms are present, but additional signs such as gaze deviation (toward the affected hemisphere), neglect, and possibly level of consciousness make this much more obvious. Therefore, the most likely explanation for the clinical picture of this patient is involvement of one or more cortical branches of the right middle cerebral artery.

Common sources of embolism include the heart, aortic arch, internal carotid artery, or the intracranial middle cerebral artery. It is often impossible to make the distinction without supporting imaging studies. However, in this case, details from the patient's history provide very helpful cues; the patient reports two prior similar episodes of left arm and face weakness that suggest recurrent ischemia in the left middle cerebral artery territory. These episodes suggest a fixed vascular lesion that is functioning as a donor site of arterial emboli, but this still does not differentiate between the middle cerebral and the internal carotid arteries. The episode of right eye visual loss is the key factor. What the patient describes is very likely an episode of amaurosis fugax and, in conjunction with the right-hemisphere symptoms, strongly suggests a stenotic atherosclerotic lesion in the extracranial internal carotid artery. Indeed, an 80% stenosis of the right proximal internal carotid artery is confirmed by CT angiography (Figure 19.1a) and is corroborated by carotid ultrasound. Brain MRI confirms acute infarcts within the right middle cerebral artery territory, as expected given the clinical presentation (Figure 19.1b). Based on the degree of vessel stenosis, the recurrent transient ischemic attacks, and now ischemic stroke, revascularization with carotid endarterectomy or carotid stenting is recommended for this symptomatic lesion. The patient is already on an optimal medical regimen and has quit smoking; therefore, it is unlikely that medical intervention only will offer sufficient long-term protection from a future, possibly disabling stroke.

Carotid stenosis was first identified as a stroke cause by Fisher during the 1950s. Our understanding of the pathophysiology of carotid atherosclerosis and its relation to cerebrovascular disease have evolved, especially since the 1990s, with several large trials evaluating the efficacy of medical and invasive interventions. The heterogeneity of these studies, the wealth of data generated, and the significant differences in individual patient characteristics make a one-size-fits-all approach impossible, although some specific conclusions seem well established. For symptomatic carotid disease with a degree of stenosis exceeding 70% and a reasonably low periprocedural risk, revascularization is recommended. The choice of carotid endarterectomy versus carotid stenting should be individualized and depends on several factors, including neck and vascular anatomy, operator experience, and comorbidities. Antiplatelet coverage with aspirin, clopidogrel, or a combination of aspirin and dipyridamole, and optimization of the rest of vascular risk factors constitute the mainstay of medical management. Unless there are specific contraindications, delaying the intervention beyond 2 weeks, as was customary in the past, does not confer any benefit.

Ideally, each patient should be approached individually, and treatment should consider age, functional status, life expectancy, comorbidities, degree of stenosis, vascular anatomy, as well as the surgeon's experience and complication rate.

(a)

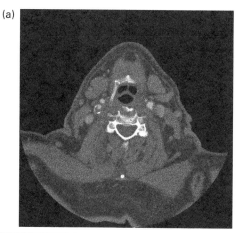

(b)

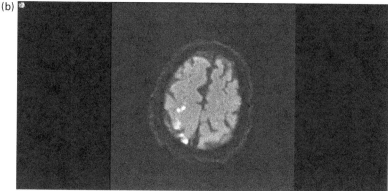

FIGURE 19.1 (a) CT angiogram of the neck showing stenosis of the proximal right internal carotid artery. (b) Diffusion-weighted MRI showing acute infarctions within the right middle cerebral artery territory.

KEY POINTS TO REMEMBER

· Recurrent symptoms of hemispheric ischemia with amaurosis fugax in the ipsilateral eye should raise concern for carotid stenosis ipsilateral to the affected hemisphere.

· Revascularization with either carotid endarterectomy or carotid stenting should be considered in patients with symptomatic lesions with more than a 70% degree of stenosis.

- Management of comorbid risk factors and lifestyle modifications are key factors in preventing stroke recurrence.
- Choice of the revascularization method (carotid endarterectomy vs. carotid stenting) should be individualized.
- Results from large trials should always be interpreted within the context of the characteristics of the population studied and the medical treatment available at the time.

Further Reading

Bonati LH, Dobson J, Featherstone RL, et al. Long-term outcomes after stenting versus endarterectomy for treatment of symptomatic carotid stenosis: the International Carotid Stenting Study (ICSS) randomised trial. *Lancet*. 2015;385(9967):529–538.

Brott TG, Halperin JL, Abbara SASA/ACCF/AHA/AANN/AANS/ACR/ASNR/CNS/SAIP/SCAI/SIR/SNIS/SVM/SVS guideline on the management of patients with extracranial carotid and vertebral artery disease: executive summary. A report of the American College of Cardiology Foundation/American Heart Association Task Force on Practice Guidelines, and the American Stroke Association, American Association of Neuroscience Nurses, American Association of Neurological Surgeons, American College of Radiology, American Society of Neuroradiology, Congress of Neurological Surgeons, Society of Atherosclerosis Imaging and Prevention, Society for Cardiovascular Angiography and Interventions, Society of Interventional Radiology, Society of NeuroInterventional Surgery, Society for Vascular Medicine, and Society for Vascular Surgery. *Circulation*. 2011;124(4):489–532.

Brott TG, Hobson RW 2nd, Howard G, Stenting versus endarterectomy for treatment of carotid-artery stenosis. *N Engl J Med*. 2010;363(1):11–23.

Kernan WN, Ovbiagele B, Black HR, et al. Guidelines for the prevention of stroke in patients with stroke and transient ischemic attack: a guideline for healthcare professionals from the American Heart Association/American Stroke Association. *Stroke*. 2014;45(7):2160–2236.

North American Symptomatic Carotid Endarterectomy Trial Collaborators. Beneficial effect of carotid endarterectomy in symptomatic patients with high-grade carotid stenosis. *N Engl J Med*. 1991;325(7):445–453.

Randomised trial of endarterectomy for recently symptomatic carotid stenosis: final results of the MRC European Carotid Surgery Trial (ECST). *Lancet*. 1998;351(9113):1379–1387.

20 "Dancing" Hand

Vasileios-Arsenios Lioutas

An 82-year-old right-handed man presents with sudden-onset movements of the right hand. He reports he woke earlier that morning in his usual state of health but he suddenly started experiencing jerky movements of his right hand, which interfered with his ability to use it. In his words: "It is as if my hand is dancing on its own." Neither his face nor any of his other limbs are affected. He has a history of hypertension for 25 years, but no history of movement disorders, and he reports no exposure to antidopaminergic agents. On examination, he is in moderate distress. He is alert and oriented, without dysarthria or language difficulties. He has no sensory deficit; his gait, coordination, and strength are intact, but his right hand is clumsy and with increased tone. There are intermittent, involuntary, abrupt, nonrhythmic movements and occasional, slow, writhing movements of the right hand that he is unable to suppress voluntarily.

What do you do now?

ACUTE FOCAL CHOREOATHETOSIS AS PRESENTATION OF ACUTE STROKE

Discussion Questions

1. What is an accurate description of this patient's symptoms?
2. What is a likely cause?
3. Are there any available treatments?

Discussion

This patient describes three different motor symptoms, two of which are hyperkinetic and one of which is hypokinetic. The jerky, nonrhythmic, involuntary hand movements could be described either as myoclonus, chorea, or hemiballismus. The range of motion and affected muscle groups are the key points in differentiating among the three. Myoclonus usually implies a rather small amplitude and affects small groups of muscle fibers whereas ballismus, on the opposite end of the spectrum, involves large, proximal muscle groups, resulting in excessive and very large range-of-motion movements. Thus, this patient's jerky "dancing" movements are best described as chorea. The second aspect of his hyperkinetic motor symptoms—the slow, writhing movements—are an accurate description of what is known as *athetosis*. Last, the hypokinetic aspect of this patient's symptoms, described as increased tone and abnormal posture of the hand, is more difficult to characterize; but, in the context of choreoathetosis, it is reasonable to assume it represents dystonia.

The abrupt onset of symptoms in a patient with long-standing hypertension and without a prior history of parkinsonism or exposure to antidopaminergic drugs suggest a possible vascular etiology. Although not widely known and often overlooked, movement disorders do occur in the context of acute stroke, either as part of the acute presentation or as a delayed manifestation. The most commonly affected areas involve the basal ganglia and the thalamus, and less frequently the brainstem. Given the complexity of the feedback circuitry among the thalamus, basal ganglia, and motor cortex that regulates movements, it is practically impossible to make accurate assumptions about lesion localization based on the nature of the motor symptoms only. For reasons that are poorly understood, hemorrhages seem to be more likely to result in a movement disorder than ischemic strokes; of the latter, small-vessel lacunar infarcts are most commonly associated with abnormal movements. This patient had, in fact, a small acute infarct in the left ventral thalamus adjacent to the area where the subthalamic nucleus is located (Figure 20.1).

Both hyperkinetic and hypokinetic movement disorders have been observed in the context of stroke. Chorea, athetosis, hemiballismus, blepharospasm, tremor, and asterixis have been described. Bradykinesia, focal or segmental dystonia, or parkinsonism have also been described. Relevant literature should be interpreted bearing in mind that the definitions of these movement disorders are, to some degree, subjective. They often present as part of acute stroke manifestations and, on some occasions, as in this case, can be the sole presenting symptom. They can cause significant distress and

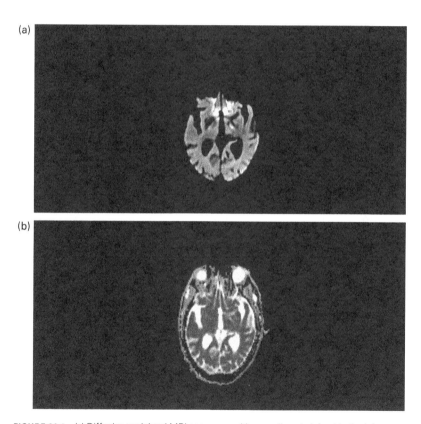

FIGURE 20.1 (a) Diffusion-weighted MRI sequence with a small acute infarct in the left subthalamic area. (b) Apparent Diffusion Coefficient (ADC) MRI sequence with corresponding hypointensity in the same area, confirming stroke acuity.

interfere with patients' daily activities; in this case, because of the involvement of his dominant hand, the patient experienced significant difficulty with feeding, and he needed supervision and help with many other tasks as well.

Several treatment options are available, depending on the nature of the motor manifestations. Typical and atypical neuroleptics, benzodiazepines, or even tetrabenazine have been tried in cases of hyperkinetic disorders such as chorea, athetosis, and ballism, with variable success. Clonazepam, baclofen, or neurotoxin injections have been used, with variable success. Poststroke tremor and parkinsonism appear refractory to medical intervention. The prognosis of stroke-related movement disorders is variable, but it seems that a majority of those (up to 65%) resolve fully or partially over time. Those that do not regress spontaneously tend to be more refractory to medical interventions, in which case a referral to a movement disorders specialist for more specialized interventions such as deep brain stimulation is reasonable.

KEY POINTS TO REMEMBER

- Movement disorders can occur in the acute or chronic phase of stroke and on occasions they can be the sole presenting clinical symptom
- Post-stroke movement disorders can take many different hyperkinetic or hypokinetic forms.
- They are relatively refractory to medical management but up to 65% of the them resolve fully or partially over time.

Further Reading

Béjot Y, Giroud M, Moreau T, Benatru I. Clinical spectrum of movement disorders after stroke in childhood and adulthood. *Eur Neurol.* 2012;68(1):59–64.

Ghika-Schmid F, Ghika J, Regli F, Bogousslavsky J. Hyperkinetic movement disorders during and after acute stroke: the Lausanne Stroke Registry. *J Neurol Sci.* 1997;146(2):109–116.

Handley A, Medcalf P, Hellier K, Dutta D. Movement disorders after stroke. *Age Ageing.* 2009;38(3):260–266.

Lee MS, Marsden CD. Movement disorders following lesions of the thalamus or subthalamic region. *Mov Disord.* 1994;9(5):493–507.

Lehéricy S, Grand S, Pollak P, et al. Clinical characteristics and topography of lesions in movement disorders due to thalamic lesions. *Neurology.* 2001;57(6):1055–1066.

21 Double Vision and Jumpy Eyes

Bart Chwalisz

A 66-year-old woman presents with sudden onset of difficulty focusing her vision and sensory changes of the left face, hand, and foot. She feels lightheaded and nauseous, and when she tries to stand she feels off-balance. She notices "blurred" vision, indicating it feels difficult to focus her eyes.

This patient has a history of poorly controlled hypertension. She takes a low-dose aspirin, hydrochlorothiazide, and losartan.

On examination she has a blood pressure of 171/80, and she is alert and conversant. There is no ptosis, and her pupils are equally reactive. Her eyes are misaligned vertically, with the left eye lower than the right. There is nystagmus in her primary gaze, with both a rotatory and a vertical component. During each half-cycle, the right eye falls and extorts while the left eye rises and intorts, then reverses on the next half-cycle. On attempted left gaze, the right eye does not adduct and the left eye displays prominent horizontal nystagmus. Convergence is intact. Gaze to the right and vertically is not impaired. Strength and reflexes are intact. Sensation is altered minimally and subjectively in the distal left hand and foot. The patient sways after standing up and holds on to the examiner's hands. Basic emergency room lab results are within normal limits, and brain CT and CT angiography of the head and neck are unremarkable.

What do you do now?

PONTINE TEGMENTUM INFARCTION WITH INTERNUCLEAR OPHTHALMOPLEGIA

Discussion Question

1. After analyzing the patient's ocular motor abnormalities, where would you localize the lesion?
2. What is the differential diagnosis?
3. What additional workup would you obtain?

Discussion

This patient presents with a complex eye movement examination but the abnormalities can be broken down into three major aspects: a vertical misalignment at rest, a vertical and rotatory nystagmus at rest, and an impairment of horizontal gaze to the right.

A vertical misalignment at rest may be the result of weakness of any one of the four muscles that move the eyes vertically (the superior and inferior recti, and the superior and inferior obliques), impairment of the innervation of these muscles, or a skew deviation. The latter is caused by unequal graviceptive vestibular input from the otolith organs of the inner ear and vestibular nuclei. In the context of brain disease, skew deviation is more common than a direct impairment of eye movement control and, conversely, it almost always indicates a central rather than a peripheral lesion, because a skew deviation results only very rarely from vestibular nerve or inner ear dysfunction. There is some localizing value to the skew deviation; the graviceptive pathway enters the brainstem in the vestibular nerve at the pontomedullary junction and decussates shortly thereafter. Because of this anatomic arrangement, the lower eye is ipsilateral to the lesion in pontomedullary lesions and contralateral to the lesion if the problem is in the pons or higher.

In addition to the misalignment of the eyes, there was nystagmus at rest—a repetitive "jerking" of the eyes, with an alternating pattern during each hemicycle—a seesaw nystagmus. Acquired nystagmus in primary gaze at rest is usually the result of disruption of the central or peripheral vestibular pathways. Peripheral vestibular nystagmus (as seen, for instance, in vestibular neuronitis) is very characteristic; it is a primarily horizontal or horizontal–torsional nystagmus that worsens with gaze toward the unaffected side and there is disruption of visual fixation. For practical purposes, almost all other forms of acquired nystagmus in primary gaze strongly suggest a central lesion in the brainstem or cerebellum. In the case of this patient, the fact that the nystagmus persisted unabated even with eyes open, and its vertical–torsional directionality, point toward a central lesion.

Last, this patient has difficulty with adducting the right eye when looking to the left. There are no other signs of oculomotor nerve dysfunction and she is able to adduct that eye with convergence. Therefore, the problem must be intranuclear (i.e., resulting from a disruption in the communication between the horizontal gaze command center for looking to the left, and the right medial rectus)—an internuclear ophthalmoplegia (INO). The final common pathway for horizontal gaze essentially originates within the abducens nucleus in the pons. It crosses the midline and communicates with the contralateral medial rectus subnucleus of the oculomotor nerve via the medial longitudinal fasciculus in the dorsal tegmentum.

Based on the patient's eye movement abnormalities, we can state that the right INO localizes to the tegmentum of the right pons or midbrain above the level of the abducens nucleus. The skew deviation with left eye hypotropia also localizes to the brainstem tegmentum; but, without the additional signs such as the INO, we would not be able to assign right or left laterality. In the current context, it also localizes to the right pontomesencephalic tegmentum. The seesaw nystagmus is a sign of brainstem dysfunction but, practically, does not allow us to refine the localization further. The mild sensory symptoms of the face, arm, and leg suggest some involvement of the sensory pathways above the level of the trigeminal nerve on the right. The patient also has some ataxia, especially of her gait. The most parsimonious hypothesis is that a single lesion in the dorsal pontine or lower midbrain tegmentum could account for all the patient's findings. Indeed, brain MRI revealed a small, right pontine tegmentum acute infarct (Figure 21.1) that, in light of the patient's poorly controlled hypertension and no other explanation from the workup, is very likely a result of small-vessel disease.

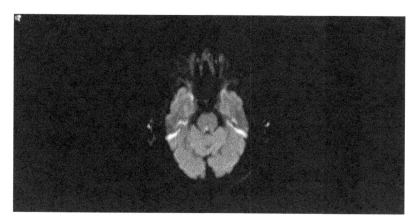

FIGURE 21.1 Diffusion-weighted MRI with a small infarct in the right posterolateral pons.

- Vertical misalignment of the eyes may be the result of either peripheral or central causes. In a patient with central nervous system pathology, skew deviation is likely to be the most common cause.
- Peripheral vestibular nystagmus is a horizontal or horizontal–torsional nystagmus that worsens with gaze toward the unaffected side and there is disruption of visual fixation. For practical purposes, all other forms of acquired nystagmus are likely to be the result of a central lesion.
- In an acutely vertiginous patient, both a nystagmus that is not clearly vestibular and the presence of skew deviation indicate a likely central lesion.
- Internuclear ophthalmoplegia (impaired adduction when looking to the opposite side, but intact convergence) is a valuable localizing sign for pontine pathology (although it can occasionally be mimicked by myasthenia gravis).
- Unilateral INO is usually the result of an infarct. Bilateral INO is most commonly caused by multiple sclerosis (but can be caused by stroke and many other pathologic processes).

Further Reading

Brodsky MC, Donahue SP, Vaphiades M, Brandt T. Skew deviation revisited. *Surv Ophthalmol*. 2006;51(2):105–128.

Eggenberger E, Golnik K, Lee A, et al. Prognosis of ischemic internuclear ophthalmoplegia. *Ophthalmology*. 2002;109:1676–1678.

Kattah JC, Talkad AV, Wang DZ, Hsieh Y-H. HINTS to diagnose stroke in the acute vestibular syndrome: three-step bedside oculomotor examination more sensitive than early MRI diffusion-weighted imaging. *Stroke*. 2009;40:3504–3510.

Kim JS. Internuclear ophthalmoplegia as an isolated or predominant symptom of brainstem infarction. *Neurology*. 2004;62:1491–1496.

Oh K, Chang JH, Park K-W, et al. Jerky seesaw nystagmus in isolated internuclear ophthalmoplegia from focal pontine lesion. *Neurology*. 2005;64:1313–1314.

22 Between a Rock and a Hard Place

Vasileios-Arsenios Lioutas

A 43-year-old right-handed man is brought to the
emergency room after being found disoriented in
his bed by his roommate. He is not in a position
to provide a reliable history, but his roommate
reports the patient has no known medical problems
and takes no medications. On examination, his
temperature is 103.2°F, he has a sinus tachycardia
with a rate of 88, and his blood pressure is 128/65.
He is agitated and combative, with mild dysarthria.
He is oriented to self, but not to time or place. He
does not seem to blink to visual threat on the right
visual field but does so on the left. He moves all
his extremities spontaneously except for his right
arm, which is flaccidly plegic, and his left leg,
which is pale and slightly colder on palpation, and
he withdraws slightly to noxious stimulation. His
language cannot be assessed in detail because
of his mental status. No meningismus is seen.

A diastolic decrescendo murmur is heard in the left parasternal border. The laboratory workup reveals a white blood cell count of 17,000, platelets of 60,000, normal renal function, and an erythrocyte sedimentation rate of 112.

What do you do now?

STROKE AND SYSTEMIC EMBOLISM RESULTING FROM BACTERIAL ENDOCARDITIS

Discussion Questions

1. What is the likely underlying cause of this patient's presentation?
2. What additional workup would you obtain?
3. How would you manage this patient?

Discussion

This patient presents with fever, leukocytosis, encephalopathy, and focal neurological deficit. An infectious process is a logical immediate consideration. Meningitis, meningoencephalitis, and intracerebral abscess are all likely causes. His lack of meningismus makes a meningitic process less likely. Encephalitis or abscess is more likely. Despite the lack of historical details, additional features in this patient's examination are helpful in furthering the diagnostic considerations. His cardiac examination, with a left parasternal border diastolic decrescendo murmur, suggests aortic regurgitation; his pulseless, pale, cold left leg suggests acute arterial embolization, which in combination with all the preceding symptoms raises concern for acute infective endocarditis resulting in arterial emboli in the brain and leg.

In this particular case, the following diagnostic tests should be considered: (1) bacterial blood cultures, ideally more than the standard two bottles, to maximize the possibility that the causative organism is identified; and (2) electrocardiogram and echocardiogram to assess cardiac function. The clinical picture suggests endocarditis of a native aortic valve without hemodynamic repercussions at the moment, but the specifics of valve function, such as vegetation size and exact location, presence of a paravalvular leak, ejection fraction, and possible involvement of additional valves, are very important in subsequent management. Transthoracic echocardiography might not be enough and often needs to be supplemented by a transesophageal test. The arterial supply to the left leg should be assessed emergently. The patient's renal function allows for use of intravenous contrast; therefore, CT or conventional angiography are ideal to identify the exact location of the arterial embolus and to guide interventions. Last, cerebral imaging should be obtained. Ideally, both the vasculature and the brain parenchyma should be assessed. Information offered by noncontrast brain CT, which is the most common imaging modality performed emergently, has inherent limitations. It does not allow for detection of acute ischemic strokes, especially of small size, and although it might detect gross intraparenchymal hemorrhage, smaller cerebral microbleeds—which are a significant feature in further anticoagulant management—cannot be detected. Intraparenchymal abscess is often difficult to differentiate from an ischemic infarct in noncontrast head CT. For all these reasons, brain MRI, ideally with contrast, is a high-yield test. Infective endocarditis leads to mycotic aneurysm formation; therefore, vessel imaging—either with CT or MR angiography—should be pursued.

In this case, vessel imaging of the leg revealed a left common femoral artery occlusion; adequate perfusion was restored with emergent thrombectomy. Although the transthoracic echocardiogram did not reveal any valvular abnormality besides mild aortic regurgitation, a transesophageal study revealed a 2 × 4-mm aortic valve vegetation. The patient's brain MRI, shown in Figure 22.1a, revealed multifocal acute infarcts—the largest being in the left frontotemporal subcortical area—with a considerable amount of a hemorrhagic component, as shown in the gradient echo sequences in Figure 22.1b. Notice that, although large hypodensities in the noncontrast head CT correspond to the ischemic infarct, the hemorrhagic component is not seen, highlighting the additional benefit of MRI in this domain.

Broad-spectrum intravenous antibiotics should be started and tailored to the identified pathogenic organism. Anticoagulation in native valve infective endocarditis is a complicated, thorny issue. Relevant literature is affected by "consultation bias" in the sense that there is a different perspective in the neurological literature, where naturally there is an overrepresentation of patients with stroke and complications, whereas in the cardiologic or infectious disease literature, a broader spectrum or presentation is seen, often leading to different perspectives. Intracerebral hemorrhage can occur via several mechanisms in patients with infective endocarditis, including hemorrhagic transformation of an ischemic stroke, rupture of a mycotic aneurysm, or erosion of a vessel wall resulting from an inflammatory vasculitic process. The first of these three mechanisms is the most common. It should be stated clearly there is no one-size-fits-all treatment and the

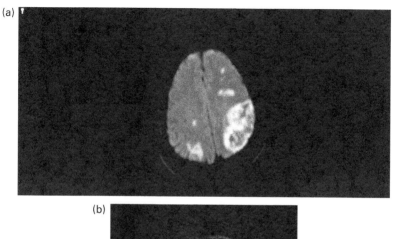

(a)

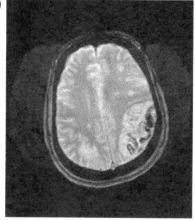

(b)

FIGURE 22.1 (a) Diffusion-weighted MRI sequence with multiple acute infarcts, with the largest affecting the left occipital lobe. (b) Gradient echo MRI sequence demonstrating blood products (dark, hypointense areas) within the acute infarct.

decision should be strictly individualized. Several factors affect the risk of both embolic and hemorrhagic complications, including age, affected valve, pathogenic organism, vegetation size, presence of mycotic aneurysm, microbleeds or overt intracerebral hemorrhage, size of ischemic stroke, other embolic complications, and urgency of possible surgical valve correction. In general, in patients with large ischemic strokes, microbleeds, or hemorrhagic conversion, mycotic aneurysms have a substantial risk of intracerebral hemorrhage, and use of antithrombotic drugs should be avoided.

· Cerebrovascular complications of bacterial infective endocarditis include ischemic stroke, mycotic aneurysm formation, inflammatory changes in the vessel wall, cerebral microbleeds, and overt intracerebral hemorrhage.

· Comprehensive brain imaging, ideally with brain MRI and including assessment of the vessels, should be performed in patients with infective endocarditis with neurological manifestations.

· Use of antithrombotic drugs in patients with infective endocarditis and stroke carries a significant intracerebral hemorrhage risk; it should be avoided if possible.

Further Reading

Cahill TJ, Prendergast BD. Infective endocarditis. *Lancet*. 2015.

Derex L, Bonnefoy E, Delahaye F. Impact of stroke on therapeutic decision making in infective endocarditis. *J Neurol*. 2010;257(3):315–321.

Ferro JM, Fonseca AC. Infective endocarditis. *Handb Clin Neurol*. 2014;119:75–91.

Hoen B, Duval X. Clinical practice: infective endocarditis. *N Engl J Med*. 2013;368(15):1425–1433.

Rasmussen RV. Anticoagulation in patients with stroke with infective endocarditis is safe. *Stroke*. 2011;42(6):1795–1796.

Sila C. Anticoagulation should not be used in most patients with stroke with infective endocarditis. *Stroke*. 2011;42(6):1797–1798.

Vilacosta I, Graupner C, San Román JA, et al. Risk of embolization after institution of antibiotic therapy for infective endocarditis. *J Am Coll Cardiol*. 2002;39(9):1489–1495.

23 Follow Your Heart or Your Brain?

Vasileios-Arsenios Lioutas

A 79-year-old right-handed man presents for
elective cardiac catheterization. He has a history
of hypertension, hyperlipidemia, diabetes,
and unstable angina. His catheterization is
uncomplicated; two-vessel disease is identified
and a drug-eluting stent is placed in the left
circumflex artery with recommendation for dual
antiplatelet coverage with aspirin and clopidogrel
for 12 months. Shortly after the procedure the
patient develops weakness of the left face, arm, and
leg, and dysarthria. On examination, he has a blood
pressure of 158/82 and an irregular heart rhythm,
with a rate of 96. He denies chest pain or dyspnea,
he is oriented to self and place but not time. He
has a left homonymous hemianopsia, with gaze
deviation to the right and neglect of his left side.
His left arm and leg are plegic, and he has complete
sensory loss in his left face, arm, and leg.

An electrocardiogram does not reveal any signs of acute cardiac ischemia and confirms the patient is in atrial fibrillation. His basic laboratory workup reveals normal renal function, an expected mild postprocedural troponin leak, red blood cell and platelet counts within normal limits, and an elevated partial thromboplastin time of 59, presumably a result of the intravenous heparin administered during the procedure.

What do you do now?

ATRIAL FIBRILLATION-RELATED STROKE IN
A PATIENT WITH RECENT MYOCARDIAL INFARCTION
WITH STENT PLACEMENT

Discussion Questions

1. What is the appropriate immediate management of this patient?
2. What are possible causes of his clinical presentation?
3. What is your long-term management plan?

Discussion

This patient's clinical presentation with dense left hemiplegia, hemianopsia, and hemihypesthesia; and profound neglect and gaze deviation suggests a large right-hemispheric lesion. Although the presence of coronary artery disease and the atrial fibrillation might lead instinctively to the thought of ischemic stroke, intracerebral hemorrhage should be considered because the patient has risk factors for it and has had intravenous heparin administered recently. Head CT should be obtained emergently. Based on the severity of his symptoms, if the patient indeed has an ischemic infarct, a proximal large-vessel occlusion is likely. Therefore, vessel imaging should be performed promptly as well, if possible, because it might offer useful information to guide subsequent management.

Urgent head CT and CT angiography of the head and neck were performed. No intracerebral hemorrhage was seen, but a right parieto-occipital hypodensity was noted, suggesting an ongoing ischemic process. The CT angiogram confirmed a complete, right proximal middle cerebral artery occlusion. Given the timing of symptom onset less than 3 hours previously, the patient should be considered for reperfusion therapies. Intravenous tissue plasminogen activator is contraindicated because of exposure to intravenous heparin and an elevated partial thromboplastin time, which increases the risk for symptomatic hemorrhage significantly if thrombolysis is administered. However, given a documented proximal middle cerebral artery occlusion, endovascular intervention can be considered and offered as an option to the patient and family. Despite several negative clinical trials in the past, five recent clinical trials have demonstrated a definitive benefit from endovascular intervention versus tissue plasminogen activator alone in patients with proximal middle cerebral artery occlusion within

6 hours from symptom onset, and therefore it should be offered, if available. In some occasions, such as in the case discussed here, endovascular intervention might be the only available treatment option. The evidence suggests the patients who benefit most from reperfusion therapies are those with good collateral circulation and those with a large "mismatch" between hypoperfused but salvageable tissue and a smaller core of irreversibly damaged tissue. In this patient's case, the hypodense area in the right parieto-temporal junction probably represents irreversible ischemia, but the severity of the clinical deficit suggests a much larger area of involved tissue that could be salvaged if that tissue is reperfused in a timely fashion.

The patient underwent an endovascular intervention with successful recanalization of the distal middle cerebral artery branches with modest, immediate postprocedural clinical improvement. The cause of his extensive infarct was not entirely clear but, given the presence of atrial fibrillation, made cardioembolism the most likely cause. An echocardiogram excluded the presence of intracardiac thrombus or valvular abnormality. Mobilization of aortic arch atherosclerotic material in the context of aortic instrumentation is another plausible mechanism of embolization, but neither the echocardiogram nor the CT angiogram revealed significant aortic arch atheroma. Therefore, atrial fibrillation is the most likely culprit.

The patient continues to be in atrial fibrillation and the issues of long-term management and secondary prevention arise. Because of the drug-eluting stent placement, dual antiplatelet coverage for 12 months is recommended by the cardiology team. Given the presence of atrial fibrillation, anticoagulation for secondary stroke prevention is also indicated, which creates a management conundrum that is not easy to address. Dual antiplatelet therapy is not generally recommended as a long-term option for secondary stroke prevention because the benefit is negated or outweighed by an increase in hemorrhagic complications. A large study addressing the safety and efficacy of combined aspirin and clopidogrel versus aspirin alone in a population of patients with atrial fibrillation corroborated this. The addition of warfarin to a regimen of aspirin and clopidogrel naturally increases the hemorrhagic risk even more. A trial conducted in Europe tested the safety of a triple regimen of aspirin, clopidogrel, and warfarin versus warfarin and clopidogrel alone in patients with indications for long-term anticoagulation who recently underwent percutaneous cardiac intervention. The dual regimen of warfarin and clopidogrel was found to be significantly safer, without increase in thrombotic complications. The answer is not simple and straightforward, and the final decision should be made after careful discussion with the treating cardiologist, the patient, and his or her family, taking into account additional details from the individual's history and weighing the risk of thrombotic complications versus the risk of hemorrhage.

KEY POINTS TO REMEMBER

- In patients with documented proximal middle cerebral artery occlusion and substantial clinical deficit, endovascular intervention might be indicated in addition to intravenous thrombolysis. Such patients should be referred to tertiary centers with the appropriate expertise.
- Intravenous tissue plasminogen activator should be offered to all eligible patients regardless of endovascular treatment consideration.
- Long-term management of patients with concurrent coronary artery disease and stroke can be challenging because of the conflicting indications. In such cases, decisions should be individualized and made after thorough discussion including the treating cardiologist.

Further Reading

ACTIVE investigators, Connolly SJ, Pogue J, et al. Effect of clopidogrel added to aspirin in patients with atrial fibrillation. *N Engl J Med.* 2009;360(20):2066–2078.

Dewilde WJ, Oirbans T, Verheugt FW, et al. Use of clopidogrel with or without aspirin in patients taking oral anticoagulant therapy and undergoing percutaneous coronary intervention: an open-label, randomised, controlled trial. *Lancet.* 2013;381(9872):1107–1115.

Jauch EC, Saver JL, Adams HP et al. Guidelines for the early management of patients with acute ischemic stroke: a guideline for healthcare professionals from the American Heart Association/American Stroke Association. *Stroke.* 2013;44(3):870–947.

Kernan WN, Ovbiagele B, Black HR et al. Guidelines for the prevention of stroke in patients with stroke and transient ischemic attack: a guideline for healthcare professionals from the American Heart Association/American Stroke Association. *Stroke*. 2014;45(7):2160–2236.

Powers WJ, Derdeyn CP, Biller J et al. 2015 AHA/ASA focused update of the 2013 guidelines for the early management of patients with acute ischemic stroke regarding endovascular treatment: a guideline for healthcare professionals from the American Heart Association/American Stroke Association. *Stroke*. 2015 Oct;46(10):3020–3035.

24 A Bloody Mesh

Vasileios-Arsenios Lioutas

A 56-year-old right-handed man is brought to the emergency room with a vague report of altered mental status. He is somnolent and difficult to arouse, and his wife provides his history at the bedside. The patient has been having slowly progressing symptoms for the past 2 months. His first complaint was diplopia, which he described as two images on top of one another. Subsequently, he developed gait balance difficulties; he needed to hold on to things to be able walk. Two or 3 weeks later, he noticed weakness of his right arm and difficulty performing tasks with his right hand. His wife thinks these developments occurred as distinct episodes, in a stepwise fashion. For the past 3 days he has been complaining of a dull headache, has had four episodes of vomiting, and has been becoming increasingly somnolent, culminating in the visit to the emergency room.

On examination, his blood pressure is 145/76. He is afebrile. He is somnolent; he opens his eyes briefly only after a sternal rub. He has bilateral eyelid ptosis. His right pupil is reactive to light but the left one is fixed at 5 mm to both direct and indirect light stimulation. He cannot move his eyes up or down, but his horizontal eye movements are intact except for left eye adduction that is partially restricted. His has mild right arm and leg paresis and ataxia. His basic laboratory workup is unremarkable.

What do you do now?

BRAINSTEM CAVERNOUS ANGIOMA

Discussion Questions

1. Where do you localize the patient's symptoms and clinical findings?
2. Comment on the pattern of symptom progression; what is the possible underlying etiology?
3. How would you treat this patient?

Discussion

Symptoms and clinical findings can be broken down into oculomotor abnormalities, right mild hemiparesis and hemiataxia, and depressed level of consciousness. With regard to the patient's oculomotor abnormalities, his initial complaint was that of vertical diplopia and his examination revealed a complete vertical gaze palsy. Supranuclear vertical gaze palsies often, although not exclusively, result from lesions in the rostral midbrain in the area of the superior colliculus, where the vertical gaze center is located. The second notable finding is that of bilateral ptosis. The muscle responsible for eyelid opening is the levator palpebrae, which is innervated by the third nerve. More important, there is one single subnucleus responsible for this particular muscle, situated in the midline, which suggests an ongoing process in that area as opposed to isolated nerve involvement after its exit from the brainstem. The pupillary reaction to light is mediated by parasympathetic fibers originating from the Edinger-Westphal nucleus, which lies in the periaqueductal area, close to the midline and subsequently following the course of the third nerve. Therefore, the lack of pupillary reaction on the left eye suggests a lesion affecting the left third nerve or the left Edinger-Westphal nucleus. Last, there is partial left adduction weakness; this horizontal eye movement is performed by the medial rectus muscle, which is innervated by the ipsilateral third nerve. Altogether, the oculomotor abnormalities suggest a lesion in the area of the upper midbrain, affecting the midline and possibly the left side more so than the right, leading to vertical gaze palsy and partial nuclear left third nerve palsy.

Right mild hemiparesis and hemiataxia could theoretically localize anywhere along the left corticospinal tract, but taking into account the oculomotor abnormalities, they most likely suggest involvement of the left cerebral peduncle in the upper midbrain tegmentum.

A depressed level of consciousness is a poorly localizing sign on its own and the potential causes are myriad. However, in light of no overt toxic, infectious, or metabolic disturbance, the progressive worsening with headache, nausea, and vomiting suggest the possibility of increased intracranial pressure. Taking into account the focal findings analyzed previously, it is concerning for obstructive hydrocephalus at the level of the third ventricle or the aqueduct of Sylvius.

The rate and mode of symptom progression allow for some hypotheses for possible underlying causes. It seems there were at least two distinct episodes of focal neurological symptoms that persisted, suggesting lasting damage. Progressive in situ thrombosis of the basilar artery is a plausible scenario; it could lead to recurrent ischemic strokes in the area of the tip of the basilar artery, which supplies the upper midbrain and the mesencephalic/diencephalic junction, and progressive thrombosis could lead to additional strokes with resulting edema causing hydrocephalus and elevated intracranial pressure. A primary intracerebral hemorrhage is unlikely to progress in such a stepwise fashion over months. Another possible explanation is a slowly growing space-occupying lesion with distinct episodes of ischemia resulting from compression of adjacent vessels or episodes of hemorrhage within and surrounding it. Primary or metastatic central nervous system tumors—especially in the area of the pineal gland—could, theoretically, have such a course, as could a vascular malformation such as an arteriovenous malformation or a cavernous angioma.

Brain MRI revealed a large, heterogeneous lesion in the rostral and upper midbrain area obstructing the third ventricle outflow and leading to obstructive hydrocephalus. Vessel imaging is unremarkable. The "popcorn" appearance in the Fluid-Attenuated Inversion Recovery (FLAIR) sequence (Figure 24.1a) and multiple microhemorrhages seen in the gradient echo sequence (Figure 24.1b) suggest a cavernous malformation with repetitive episodes of microhemorrhage.

Cavernous malformations are known by several different terms: *cavernous angioma, cavernous hemangioma*, and *cavernoma*. They consist of a mesh of capillary vessels without intervening brain parenchyma, with

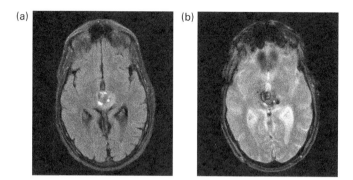

FIGURE 24.1 (a) MRI fluid-attenuated inversion recovery FLAIR sequence with the characteristic "popcorn" heterogeneous appearance. (b) Gradient echo MRI sequence with multiple microhemorrhages (dark, hypointense areas within the cavernoma).

abnormal vessel wall histology that makes them prone to blood leak and hemorrhage. They are low-vascular flow lesions, which renders them occult angiographically, even with conventional angiography, although on occasion a draining vein might be identified. Brain MRI with the characteristic popcorn appearance on T2 sequences with or without evidence of microhemorrhages is the imaging modality of choice. Most of them occur de novo, although there are familial forms linked to specific gene mutations. They can be solitary or multiple and can be found anywhere in the brain or spinal cord. A majority of them remain clinically silent and are incidental imaging findings. They might manifest clinically with seizures, focal neurological symptoms, or hemorrhage. The 5-year risk of first hemorrhage is 2.4%.

Their natural history is complex, and management often poses a significant challenge; several parameters should be taken into consideration: whether the lesion is symptomatic, size, location, and surgical accessibility. Brainstem lesions are more challenging technically and carry greater operative risk. Surgical removal is often retained as a solution for lesions that are symptomatic, and the risk of neurological complications outweighs the periprocedural complication risk. It is important that concurrent issues (such as seizures or increased intracranial pressure, in this case) be addressed promptly and that the patient be referred to a center with neurosurgeons experienced in the management of such lesions.

· Rostral midbrain lesions lead to conjugate vertical gaze abnormalities.

· Cavernous malformations can manifest with seizures, focal neurological deficits, or hemorrhages.

· Cavernous malformations are occult angiographically; they cannot be identified with vessel imaging. The imaging modality of choice is brain MRI, in which the images have a characteristic popcorn appearance in T2 sequences.

· Management of cavernous malformations is not straightforward, and the decision for surgical removal should be made carefully, weighing several different factors. Ideally, patients should be referred to neurosurgeons with experience in managing such lesions.

Further Reading

Abla AA, Turner JD, Mitha AP, Lekovic G, Spetzler RF. Surgical approaches to brainstem cavernous malformations. *Neurosurg Focus*. 2010;29(3):E8.

Al-Shahi Salman R, Hall JM, Horne MA, et al. Untreated clinical course of cerebral cavernous malformations: a prospective, population-based cohort study. *Lancet Neurol*. 2012;11(3):217–224.

Josephson CB, Leach JP, Duncan R, et al. Seizure risk from cavernous or arteriovenous malformations: prospective population-based study. *Neurology*. 2011;76(18):1548–1554.

Li D, Hao SY, Jia GJ, Wu Z, Zhang LW, Zhang JT. Hemorrhage risks and functional outcomes of untreated brainstem cavernous malformations. *J Neurosurg*. 2014;121(1):32–41.

25 A Lernaean Hydra

Vasileios-Arsenios Lioutas

A 65-year-old right-handed man presents to the
emergency room with acute onset of right-sided
face, arm, and leg weakness, and global aphasia.
Despite his dramatic, acute presentation he does
not receive intravenous thrombolysis because
of rapidly improving symptoms and a platelet
count of 58,000. Head CT is unremarkable, and CT
angiography of the head and neck reveals patent
vessels. On examination 3 hours after his initial
presentation, his only deficit is a slight right leg
weakness. His past history includes pancreatic
adenocarcinoma, hypertension, and diabetes
mellitus. His medications include 325 mg aspirin
daily, insulin, and multivitamins. No change is
noticed in subsequent half-hourly evaluations
until, 3 hours later, when an acute change is noted.
The patient has become less responsive, with a
forced gaze deviation to the right; complete plegia
of the left face, arm, and leg; left hemineglect;
and hemianopsia. His National Institutes of Health

Stroke Scale score is 17. He is afebrile, with a blood pressure of 134/67 and a sinus rhythm of 68. Despite his severe deficit, he does not recognize any problem subjectively. Repeat CT angiography reveals, this time, a proximal right middle cerebral artery (MCA) occlusion.

Besides the thrombocytopenia, his laboratory workup is notable for an international normalized ratio of 1.3, hematocrit of 34, fibrin degradation products, and d-Dimer more than 10-fold the upper level of the laboratory reference value.

What do you do now?

MULTIPLE ACUTE STROKES IN RAPID SUCCESSION RESULTING FROM CANCER-RELATED HYPERCOAGULABILITY

Discussion Questions

1. How would you treat this patient acutely?
2. What are the possible underlying causes of this patient's presentation?
3. What additional workup would you pursue?
4. What would be your management approach?

Discussion

The initial presentation of this patient suggests extensive ischemia of the left hemisphere, based on severe plegia and global aphasia. A plausible scenario is ischemia of the MCA and possibly the anterior cerebral artery (ACA), likely from an embolus in the terminal internal carotid artery or proximal MCA with spontaneous resolution. The residual, mild right-leg weakness, although not strictly localizing, suggests a relatively small residual infarct possibly in the left ACA territory. (Vascular supply to the part of the motor cortex controlling the leg is provided by the ACA.) The second event, which occurred in rapid succession, suggests significant right-hemisphere ischemia. Besides the left-sided hemiplegia and hemianopsia, the patient also has profound neglect, forced rightward gaze deviation, and anosognosia. CT angiography confirms a proximal right MCA occlusion

This patient had a substantial neurological deficit captured within minutes of its onset, which offers significant potential for improvement if treated timely. Intravenous thrombolysis is not a consideration given the thrombocytopenia, but the documented proximal MCA occlusion makes him a good candidate for endovascular intervention, if he prefers aggressive management.

This is an unusually aggressive, malignant course. The patient essentially experienced two major arterial occlusive events, presumably of embolic etiology, in different vascular territories within 3 to 4 hours of one another. It is reasonable to assume the embolic source is proximal to the origin of the brachiocephalic artery, thus explaining involvement of both the right and left MCA territories. Atrial fibrillation is naturally considered because it is a very common source of cardioembolism, but the patient neither has a history of it nor does his continuous cardiac monitor reveal any arrhythmias.

Besides, Although such an aggressive course with multiple major embolic events in rapid succession is plausible, it is not seen frequently in atrial fibrillation-associated stroke. At this point, it should be noted there are signs of a coagulopathy, with thrombocytopenia, mild elevation of the international normalized ratio, and very elevated fibrin degradation products; in light of underlying cancer, a hypercoagulable state—possibly chronic disseminated intravascular coagulation—is suspected. This could lead to intracardiac thrombus formation or recurrent paradoxical embolism from a deep vein thrombus if a patent foramen ovale is present. Non-specific malignancy-related hypercoagulability can lead to recurrent arterial thromboembolism without the presence of the previous two conditions. Malignant cancers, and especially mucin-producing adenocarcinomas, are associated with non-bacterial thrombotic endocarditis, also known as *marantic endocarditis*. As its name implies, it is characterized by formation of small, sterile vegetations in the valve leaflets, consisting primarily of fibrin and platelets but without microorganisms or inflammation. The vegetations act as nidus for further thrombus formation that can embolize distally.

Therefore, an echocardiogram and brain MRI are necessary. The echocardiogram did not reveal intracardiac thrombus or valve vegetations—corroborated by a detailed transesophageal study. Patent foramen ovale or other right-to-left shunt was not detected. Brain MRI revealed a large, right MCA territory acute stroke (Figure 25.1a), a smaller left ACA territory infarct, as well as several other scattered acute infarcts, in several different vascular territories (Figure 25.1b). In the absence of other alternative explanations and in light of the elevated d-Dimer level and increased fibrin degradation products cancer-related hypercoagulability is the most likely cause.

Ischemic stroke occurs in the context of cancer-related hypercoagulability; solid tumors and especially adenocarcinomas are the most commonly implicated cancers, predominantly pancreatic and lung. Unless there is a specific contraindication, anticoagulation is recommended for recurrent stroke prophylaxis. Although no data from high-quality trials exist, low-molecular weight heparin is preferred over warfarin. The relationship between stroke and cancer is bidirectional; stroke affects cancer patients' ability to participate in aggressive chemotherapy regimens negatively and cancer can delay stroke recovery significantly. It is therefore imperative that, before aggressive measures are taken, the severity and stage of

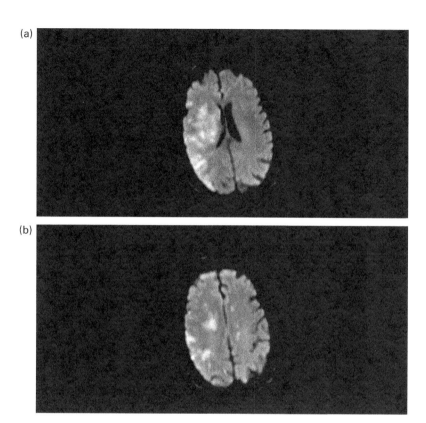

(a)

(b)

FIGURE 25.1 (a) Large, acute right-hemispheric stroke. (b) Scattered, acute bihemispheric strokes in the right middle cerebral artery and left anterior cerebral artery territories.

the underlying malignancy are taken into account. The patient and family should be informed thoroughly about prognosis, recovery, and implications of proposed treatments; with the treating oncologist involved in the decision making. This approach ensures all proposed interventions are in agreement with the patient's wishes.

Further Reading

Asopa S, Patel A, Khan OA, Sharma R, Ohri SK. Non-bacterial thrombotic endocarditis. *Eur J Cardiothorac Surg.* 2007;32(5):696–701.

Bang OY, Seok JM, Kim SG, et al. Ischemic stroke and cancer: stroke severely impacts cancer patients, while cancer increases the number of strokes. *J Clin Neurol.* 2011;7(2):53–59.

Cestari DM, Weine DM, Panageas KS, Segal AZ, DeAngelis LM. Stroke
in patients with cancer: incidence and etiology. *Neurology*.
2004;62(11):2025–2030.

Schwarzbach CJ, Schaefer A, Ebert A, et al. Stroke and cancer: the importance of
cancer-associated hypercoagulation as a possible stroke etiology. *Stroke*.
2012;43(11):3029–3034.

26 It Looks Like a Stroke, Walks Like a Stroke, and Behaves Like a Stroke. But Is It a Stroke?

Vasileios-Arsenios Lioutas

A 61-year-old right-handed woman is brought to the emergency room with confusion and right-sided weakness. She is brought in by emergency medical service personnel who were alerted by the patient's daughter; the patient was not answering her phone calls. The last communication was the night before presentation, at which point the patient was at her baseline, complaining of a moderately severe headache. The paramedical personnel report the patient was found on the floor, unable to walk, complaining of severe headache and unable to recount her history. En route to the hospital she had a brief episode of clonic activity of the right face and arm, responding to 1 mg intravenous lorazepam. On examination, she is afebrile, with a blood pressure of 191/90 and a sinus tachycardia of 92. There is no meningismus. She is alert, but is inattentive and oriented to person and year only. She is mildly dysarthric and can name and repeat without difficulty, but has difficulty following complex instructions. She has decreased blink to visual threat on the left, and a mild hemiparesis and ataxia of her right arm and, to a lesser extent, her right leg.

Her past history includes hypertension and depression. Medications include fluoxetine, started 2 months previously, and lisinopril. Basic emergency laboratory workup is notable only for increased creatinine to 1.8.

What do you do now?

POSTERIOR REVERSIBLE ENCEPHALOPATHY SYNDROME

Discussion Questions

1. What is the differential diagnosis for this patient's presentation?
2. What additional workup would you consider?
3. How would you manage this patient?

Discussion

This patient's presentation is puzzling. She has neurological deficits that suggest focal lesions: right hemiparesis and hemiataxia, left homonymous visual field cut, and an episode strongly suggestive of a focal motor seizure. Her mental state, with inattention and confusion, does not localize accurately. Careful language examination suggests there is no focal language deficit and her difficulty following complex commands is the result of inattention; patient's mental state would therefore be best described as encephalopathy. Taken into account, the findings suggest a multifocal process with acute onset. Whether the symptoms presented concurrently and abruptly or developed over several hours is not clear. Multifocal ischemic strokes—an "embolic shower" from a cardiac, arterial, or venous (through paradoxical embolism) source—are a plausible explanation, although she has no apparent risk factors predisposing her to multifocal cerebral embolism. Multifocal intracerebral hemorrhage is another consideration, especially given the headache. However, despite the patient's markedly elevated blood pressure, a known risk factor for primary intracerebral hemorrhage, simultaneously occurring multifocal hemorrhages is extremely uncommon. Hemorrhagic metastatic brain lesions are another consideration; certain malignancies have the tendency to bleed—and some of those can do so simultaneously—with melanoma being a characteristic example. Other space-occupying lesions such as primary central nervous system tumors or abscesses could also conceivably cause multifocal neurological symptoms and encephalopathy. Meningoencephalitis is another theoretical consideration, although the lack of fever, leukocytosis, and meningismus make this less likely, although it cannot be ruled out completely. Cerebral venous sinus thrombosis is another consideration in a patient with headache, encephalopathy, and focal neurological symptoms. Last, hypertensive encephalopathy and, more specifically, the syndrome known as *posterior reversible encephalopathy*, or PRES, is a consideration.

From a clinical perspective, one important additional test that should be performed is a funduscopic examination, which would not only point toward some of the previously mentioned diagnoses, but also would provide evidence for the presence or absence of papilledema, which in turn could prevent physicians from performing potentially dangerous diagnostic procedures such as lumbar puncture in the context of increased intracranial pressure. Urgent head CT can differentiate easily between a hemorrhagic and an ischemic lesion. Indeed, the head CT in this case did not reveal any hemorrhagic lesions, but hypodensities of both hemispheres, primarily in the posterior frontal and parietal and occipital areas, were noted. This finding is nonspecific and, besides ruling out hemorrhage, it leaves many of the previous questions unanswered. Brain MRI should be obtained and— given that metastatic, primary central nervous system tumors, abscesses, and other infectious processes are considered—a contrast-enhanced study should ideally be added. Vessel imaging, including both the arterial and the venous supply and drainage to the brain, should also be performed.

Magnetic resonance angiography and venography did not reveal any abnormalities. Fluid-attenuated inversion recovery (FLAIR) MRI sequences revealed extensive hyperintensities in the brain areas corresponding to the hypodensities seen in the CT scan (Figure 26.1a). Diffusion-weighted images (DWI) (Figure 26.1b) are of mixed intensity, but primarily hypointense and in combination with hyperintense apparent diffusion coefficient (ADC) (Figure 26.1c) images, strongly suggest the diagnosis of PRES in light of the clinical picture. Acute ischemia would have resulted in hyperintense DWI and hypointense ADC images.

PRES is a diagnosis identified and first described as a distinct entity in 1996, then termed *posterior reversible leukoencephalopathy syndrome*. It is a clinicoradiologic syndrome with headache, encephalopathy, visual disturbances, and often seizures. Traditionally, a predilection for the white matter posterior cerebral regions—especially the parieto-occipital lobes— has been described. However, as our understanding of the syndrome has evolved, involvement of other cerebral regions and the cortex is not unusual and, depending on the location, focal neurological symptoms are not uncommon. Brain MRI is important in establishing the diagnosis,

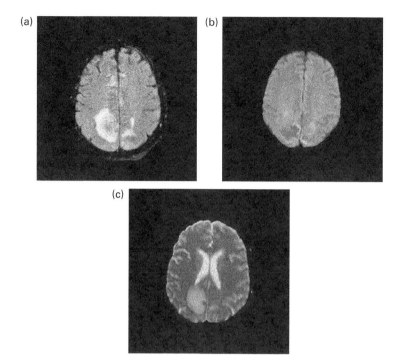

FIGURE 26.1 (a) Extensive bihemispheric FLAIR hyperintensities, predominantly posterior. (b, c) Diffusion-weighted images (DWI) and apparent diffusion coefficient (ADC) MRI sequences. Notice that, contrary to acute ischemia, the DWI are hypointense whereas ADC images are hyperintense.

with imaging characteristics of vasogenic edema as described in detail earlier, with a hemorrhagic component seen on some occasions. PRES is seen in the context of several conditions. Severe hypertension and preeclampsia/eclampsia are perhaps the best known, but it should be emphasized that PRES can be seen in normotensive patients. Allogenic bone marrow and solid organ transplantations, cancer chemotherapy, immunosuppression, systemic inflammatory response syndrome, and autoimmune conditions have all been described as predisposing factors. The pathophysiology is not well understood. Hyperperfusion and fluid extravasation have been postulated in the case of hypertension, whereas an endothelial dysfunction as a response to circulating cytokines is another proposed mechanism.

There is no specific, targeted treatment for PRES. Patients should be monitored closely and treated for underlying infectious processes, electrolyte imbalances, and seizures. Predisposing factors such as immuno-suppressants or chemotherapeutic agents should be removed at least tempo-rarily, if possible. Blood pressure should be lowered carefully in a controlled environment in those presenting with severe hypertension; aggressive con-trol leading to a precipitous drop might be harmful. Although no specific thresholds or numeric cutoffs are available, a stepwise reduction by 25% per 24 hours is a reasonable reference point. The long-term prognosis is generally favorable.

KEY POINTS TO REMEMBER

- PRES is a clinicoradiologic syndrome presenting with headache, encephalopathy, seizures, and occasionally focal neurological symptoms.
- PRES has a predilection for posterior cerebral regions but is not restricted to them and can be seen in anterior and infratentorial regions as well.
- MRI with hyperintense T2/FLAIR, hypointense DWI, and hyperintense ADC sequences can be particularly helpful in distinguishing PRES from other conditions.
- Hypertension, eclampsia, solid organ and bone marrow transplantation, chemotherapy and immunosuppression, systemic inflammatory response, and autoimmune diseases have all been linked to PRES.
- Long-term prognosis is generally favorable.

Further Reading

Bartynski WS. Posterior reversible encephalopathy syndrome, part 1: fundamental imaging and clinical features. *AJNR Am J Neuroradiol.* 2008;29(6):1036–1042.

Bartynski WS. Posterior reversible encephalopathy syndrome, part 2: controversies surrounding pathophysiology of vasogenic edema. *AJNR Am J Neuroradiol.* 2008;29(6):1043–1049.

Hinchey J, Chaves C, Appignani B, et al. A reversible posterior leukoencephalopathy syndrome. *N Engl J Med.* 1996;334(8):494–500.

Lamy C, Oppenheim C, Mas JL. Posterior reversible encephalopathy syndrome. *Handb Clin Neurol.* 2014;121:1687–1701.

Lamy C, Oppenheim C, Méder JF, Mas JL. Neuroimaging in posterior reversible encephalopathy syndrome. *J Neuroimaging*. 2004;14(2):89–96.

Roth C, Ferbert A. Posterior reversible encephalopathy syndrome: long-term follow-up. *J Neurol Neurosurg Psychiatry*. 2010;81(7):773–777.

27 A Relentless Headache

Vasileios-Arsenios Lioutas

A 63-year-old right-handed man with intense headache and right-arm numbness presents to the emergency department. He reports that his symptoms started 4 days earlier with an intense headache in his left occipital area. He describes it as the worst headache of his life. He indicates the headache reached its maximum intensity within seconds, and notes there was no associated photophobia or phonophobia, but he felt nauseous. The headache was not accompanied by other symptoms; it lasted for approximately 6 hours and subsided spontaneously. A similar headache recurred the next day, again with no accompanying neurological or other symptoms besides nausea, and it, too, resoled spontaneously over several hours. A third episode of a similar abrupt-onset, very intense, focal, headache occurred several hours previously and led the patient to seek medical attention. This time, the patient experienced a 45-minute episode of right face and arm paresthesias. He cannot elaborate further on the rate of progression of the symptoms, but currently has no symptoms besides the headache. On examination, he is afebrile and in moderate distress, with a blood pressure of 135/85 and a normal heart rate with a regular rhythm. There is no meningismus. His neurological examination, including a fundoscopic examination, does not reveal any abnormalities. He denies any recent or remote head or neck injury. He has no prior history of headache. His only medical problem is depression, for which he began taking phenelzine 6 weeks earlier. He does not consume alcohol or tobacco.

What do you do now?

REVERSIBLE CEREBRAL VASOCONSTRICTION SYNDROME

Discussion Questions

1. What is your differential diagnosis for this patient's presentation?
2. What imaging and laboratory workup would you pursue?
3. How would you treat and counsel the patient?

Discussion

This patient presented with recurrent, abrupt-onset, very intense headache; this pattern of headache presentation is known as *thunderclap*. Naturally, the first thought of a clinician hearing such as story is subarachnoid hemorrhage secondary to aneurysmal rupture. Broadening the diagnostic considerations, in a patient with lateralized headache and focal, transient neurological symptoms, complex migraine is a consideration. The patient has no prior history of migraines and the headache in migraine usually builds up over several minutes, making this a less likely scenario. Certain primary headache syndromes belonging to a group known as *trigeminal autonomic cephalalgias* present abruptly. Paroxysmal hemicrania continua, cluster headache, and short-lasting unilateral neuralgiform headache belong to this group, but it is relatively unlikely for them to present during the seventh decade of life, the patient is lacking certain characteristic autonomic features, and these headaches are not commonly associated with focal neurological symptoms in the torso and limbs. In a patient with headache or neck pain and focal neurological deficits, carotid or vertebral artery dissection should be in the differential diagnosis. The lack of neck or head injury does not necessarily rule out dissection, although it should be noted that thunderclap is a relatively uncommon pattern of pain presentation in arterial dissections. Last, a vasculitic process, either inflammatory or infectious vasculitis or reversible cerebral vasoconstriction syndrome (RCVS), are additional diagnostic considerations.

Brain CT and vessel imaging should be pursued emergently. Head CT of this patient revealed bilateral convexal subarachnoid hemorrhage in the parieto-occipital areas (Figure 27.1a). Although this steers our diagnostic thinking toward some of the conditions considered earlier (aneurysmal subarachnoid hemorrhage and RCVS), it creates an additional diagnostic conundrum. Aneurysmal rupture most commonly results in large, sulcal subarachnoid hemorrhage; therefore, a convexal location makes aneurysmal rupture less likely. However, other conditions such as cerebral amyloid angiopathy and cortical vein thrombosis can be added to the differential diagnosis.

CT and conventional angiography confirm the presence of diffuse vasospasm (Figure 27.1b), and brain MRI is free of cortical or subcortical microbleeds. Therefore, the most likely diagnosis for this patient is RCVS.

RCVS is a clinicoradiologic syndrome known in the past under many different names, such as *postpartum angiitis* (as a result of the fact that it was seen more frequently and identified erroneously as a purely postpartum condition) or *Call-Fleming syndrome*. It is characterized by recurrent thunderclap headaches with or without focal neurological symptoms. Neuroimaging is crucial in establishing the diagnosis and excluding alternative explanations. Subarachnoid blood is not uncommon. As mentioned earlier, RCVS takes the form of convexal hemorrhage as opposed to aneurysmal subarachnoid hemorrhage, where blood can be seen in the Sylvian fissure and the basal cisterns. Vessel imaging confirms the presence of diffuse vasospasm and excludes the presence of aneurysm. Conventional angiography remains the gold standard, but magnetic resonance or CT angiography are often sufficient. It should be emphasized that the angiographic detection of vasospasm depends on the timing of vessel imaging; if performed too early, vasospasm might be missed. This implies there might be a discrepancy between clinical presentation and angiographic appearance. Similarly, angiography is useful in establishing reversal of vasoconstriction; exactly when this occurs is not well established, but in general it is expected to resolve within the first few weeks of presentation. Persistent vessel changes should raise concern for alternative diagnoses. A common diagnostic dilemma is RCVS versus primary angiitis of the central nervous system. The latter is, in fact, rather rare and its clinical presentation is markedly different. It is characterized by more long-standing vague headaches and persistent neurological symptoms, and the angiographic appearance might be quite different, with persistent vessel wall changes, including focal dilatations. Although cerebrospinal fluid analysis is not always performed as part of an RVCS workup, it should be performed if primary angiitis is considered, in which case it reveals an inflammatory profile.

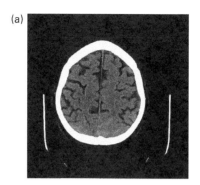

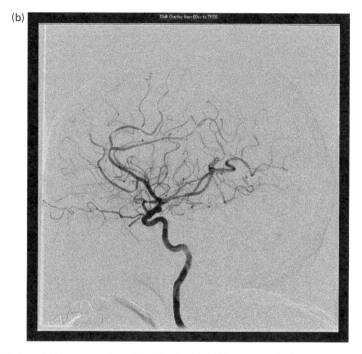

FIGURE 27.1   (a) Noncontrast head CT with subarachnoid hemorrhage in the parieto-occipital convexity bilaterally. (b) Conventional angiogram (injection of the right internal carotid artery) with multiple areas of "beading," "sausage-shaped" areas of arterial constriction.

The etiology of RCVS is not well known. It has been associated with vasoactive drugs, including nasal decongestants, selective serotonin reuptake inhibitors, triptans, monoamine oxidase inhibitors (as is phenelzine in this patient), or recreational drug use such as cocaine. It has also been seen in the peripartum period (hence the term *postpartum angiitis*) and during intense physical exercise. Calcium channel blockers are the usual agent of choice for management because of their vasodilatory capacity. Verapamil is an agent commonly chosen; it should be emphasized there is no specific indication for nimodipine in RCVS, contrary to vasospasm following aneurysmal subarachnoid hemorrhage.

The long-term prognosis is generally favorable in the sense that the majority of patients survive without neurological deficits. Chronic headache necessitating long-term management and more vague complaints such as dizziness and fatigue are not uncommon, and in that sense the quality of life of some RCVS patients is affected negatively.

KEY POINTS TO REMEMBER

· RCVS is a clinicoradiologic syndrome with a clinical presentation of thunderclap headache, with or without focal neurological deficits

· Convexal subarachnoid hemorrhage is a common imaging finding.

· The exact etiology of RCVS is not known, but it is associated with exposure to sympathomimetic, vasoactive substances; puerperium; and vigorous physical exercise.

· Vessel imaging reveals diffuse vasoconstriction, which reverses within a few weeks of presentation.

· Calcium channel blockers are often used for symptomatic management.

· The long-term prognosis is generally favorable, although residual chronic headaches are not uncommon.

Further Reading

Beitzke M, Gattringer T, Enzinger C, Wagner G, Niederkorn K, Fazekas F. Clinical presentation, etiology, and long-term prognosis in patients with nontraumatic convexal subarachnoid hemorrhage. *Stroke*. 2011;42(11):3055–3060.

John S, Singhal AB, Calabrese L, et al. Long-term outcomes after reversible cerebral vasoconstriction syndrome. *Cephalalgia*. 2015. pii: 0333102415591507. [Epub ahead of print]

Kumar S, Goddeau RP Jr, Selim MH, et al. Atraumatic convexal subarachnoid hemorrhage: clinical presentation, imaging patterns, and etiologies. *Neurology*. 2010;74(11):893–899.

Marder CP, Narla V, Fink JR, Tozer Fink KR. Subarachnoid hemorrhage: beyond aneurysms. *AJR Am J Roentgenol*. 2014;202(1):25–37.

Singhal AB, Hajj-Ali RA, Topcuoglu MA, et al. Reversible cerebral vasoconstriction syndromes: analysis of 139 cases. *Arch Neurol*. 2011;68(8):1005–1012.

Whyte CA, Calabrese LH. Reversible cerebral vasoconstriction syndrome. *Headache*. 2009;49(4):597–598.

Index

Page numbers followed by *f* indicate figures and those followed by *t* indicate tables.

in alexia without agraphia in young
woman with complex migraines
management, 91
in atrial fibrillation–related stroke in
patient with recent myocardial
infarction with stent placement
management, 136–137
in Eagle's syndrome management, 72
in recurrent ischemic strokes
resulting from ICAD
management, 97
in symptomatic right internal carotid
artery stenosis management, 114
ataxia(s)
after lifting vacuum cleaner, 19–25,
23f, 22f (*see also* lateral medullary
syndrome, nontraumatic
dissection and)
gastroenteritis with, 63–68, 66f (*see also*
cerebellar infarct)
atherosclerosis
carotid
pathophysiology of, 114
atherosclerotic dolichoectasia, 54
athetosis
described, 118
atrial fibrillation
paroxysmal
cardioembolism from, 95
atrial fibrillation–related stroke
in patient with recent myocardial
infarction with stent placement,
133–138
evaluation of, 133–135
imaging studies of, 135–136
long-term management and
secondary prevention in, 136–137
presentation of, 133–135
treatment of, 136–137
aura(s)
migraine with (*see* migraine with aura)
migrainous visual, 89
Avakame, E., 45

bacterial endocarditis
ICH due to, 130–131
stroke and systemic embolism from,
127–132, 131f
complications of, 130–131
imaging studies of, 129–131, 131f
presentation of, 127–129
treatment of, 130–131
workup for, 127–129
Beth Israel Deaconess Medical Neurology
Department, viii
bias(es)
"consultation," 130
bilateral ptosis, 141
blindness
transient monocular, 57–62, 61f
(*see also* transient monocular
visual loss (TMVL))
blood hyperviscosity
cerebellar infarct from, 63–68, 66f
(*see also* cerebellar infarct)
blood pressure
elevated
lateral medullary syndrome
and, 19–20
increased
malignant MCA infarct and, 14
lowering of
in lobar ICH from amyloid
angiopathy management, 5
"blurred" vision, 121–126, 125f
blurry vision, 57–62, 61f. *see also*
transient monocular visual
loss (TMVL)
body weakness
eyelid droopiness and, 99–104,
102f (*see also* Horner's
syndrome; right carotid
artery dissection)
border-zone infarcts
hypoperfusion-related ischemia leading
to, 97, 96
Bouffard, M., 19

deep vein thrombosis
  malignant MCA infarct and, 14
Dejerine–Roussy syndrome, 108
Dejerine syndrome, 45–50, 48*f*
depression
  cortical spreading, 89
diet
  in ICAD management, 97
digital subtraction angiography
  after Eagle's syndrome, 72
diplopia
  vertical, 141, 139
dipyridamole
  in symptomatic right internal
    carotid artery stenosis
    management, 114
distal arterial embolism
  recurrent ischemic strokes due
    to, 97, 96
dizziness
  after lifting vacuum cleaner, 19–25,
    23*f*, 22*f* (*see also* lateral medullary
    syndrome, nontraumatic
    dissection and)
  described, 63
  gastroenteritis with, 63–68, 66*f* (*see also*
    cerebellar infarct)
  twisted tongue and, 45–50, 48*f* (*see also*
    medial medullary infarct)
dolichoectasia
  atherosclerotic, 54
  causes of, 54
  congenital, 54
  described, 54
  diseases predisposing to, 54–55
  imaging studies of, 53, 54*f*
  presentation of, 51–53
  prognosis of, 56
  stroke after
    mechanisms of, 55
  treatment of, 55
  vertebrobasilar, 53–56, 54*f*
double vision

jumpy eyes and, 121–126, 125*f* (*see*
    also internuclear ophthalmoplegia
    (INO), pontine tegmentum
    infarction with)
  sudden onset of
    with left ataxic hemiparesis,
      75–80, 78*f*, 77*f* (*see also* rostral
      mesencephalic–medial thalamic
      stroke syndrome)
dysarthria, 45–50, 48*f*. *see also* medial
    medullary infarct

Eagle's syndrome
  causes of, 71
  described, 73
  digital subtraction angiography after, 72
  forms of, 73
  imaging studies of, 71, 72*f*
  internal carotid artery dissection
    and stroke complicating,
    69–74, 72*f*
    long-term stroke prevention in
      management of, 72
    presentation of, 69–71
    treatment of, 71–73
  laboratory studies of, 71
  symptoms of, 69–71
Eagle, W., 73
echocardiogram
  for multiple acute strokes in rapid
    succession due to cancer-related
    hypercoagulability, 148
edema
  brain
    CVST with, 81–85, 83*f* (*see also*
      cerebral venous sinus thrombosis
      (CVST), with hemorrhage and
      brain edema)
Edinger-Westphal nucleus, 141
elongated styloid process
  compression of extracranial carotid
    artery by, 73
"embolic shower," 153

ICAD and, 93–98, 96*f* (*see also*
        intracranial atherosclerotic disease
        (ICAD), recurrent ischemic strokes
        resulting from)
    migraine aura *vs.*, 90–91
    in posterior circulation
        vertigo suggestive of, 47
    stroke following, 53–56, 54*f*
transient monocular blindness, 57–62, 61*f.*
        see also transient monocular visual
        loss (TMVL)
transient monocular visual loss (TMVL)
    carotid stenosis causing, 57–62, 61*f*
        presentation of, 57–59
    causes of, 59–62, 61*f*
    diagnosis of, 60
    imaging studies of, 61, 60
    laboratory testing for, 60
    treatment of, 60–61
tremor(s)
    cerebellar infarct and, 65
    rubral, 79
trigeminal autonomic cephalgias, 161
twisted tongue
    dizziness and, 45–50, 48*f* (*see also*
        medial medullary infarct)

ultrasound
    for recurrent ischemic strokes resulting
        from ICAD, 96

vacuum cleaner
    lifting of
        dizziness and ataxia after, 19–25,
        23*f,* 22*f* (*see also* lateral medullary
        syndrome, nontraumatic
        dissection and)
Van Nostrand, M., 33
vascular imaging
    for TMVL, 60
vasoactive drugs
    RCVS related to, 163
venography

CT
    for CVST, 10
    magnetic resonance
        for CVST, 9, 83, 10
        for PRES, 154
vertebral artery
    left
        occlusive dissection of, 22–24, 23*f*
vertebrobasilar dolichoectasia, 53–56, 54*f.*
        see also dolichoectasia
vertical diplopia, 141, 139
vertical misalignment of eyes at rest
    of eyes, 123
vertigo
    headache and, 45–50, 48*f* (*see also*
        medial medullary infarct)
    lightheadedness and, 63
    room-spinning
        sudden onset of, 19
    suggestive of posterior circulation stroke
        or TIA in posterior circulation, 47
    for 24 hours, 19
vessel imaging
    for RCVS, 162
vision
    "blurred," 121–126, 125*f*
    blurry, 57–62, 61*f* (*see also* transient
        monocular visual loss (TMVL))
    double (*see* double vision)
    "graying of," 57
visual disturbances
    in young woman with complex
        migraines, 87
visual loss
    transient monocular
        carotid stenosis causing, 57–62, 61*f*
        (*see also* transient monocular visual
        loss (TMVL))
vitamin K
    in hypertensive primary ICH
        management, 42
vitamin K antagonists
    in CVST management, 10